# LONE
# W·O·L·F

T0346512

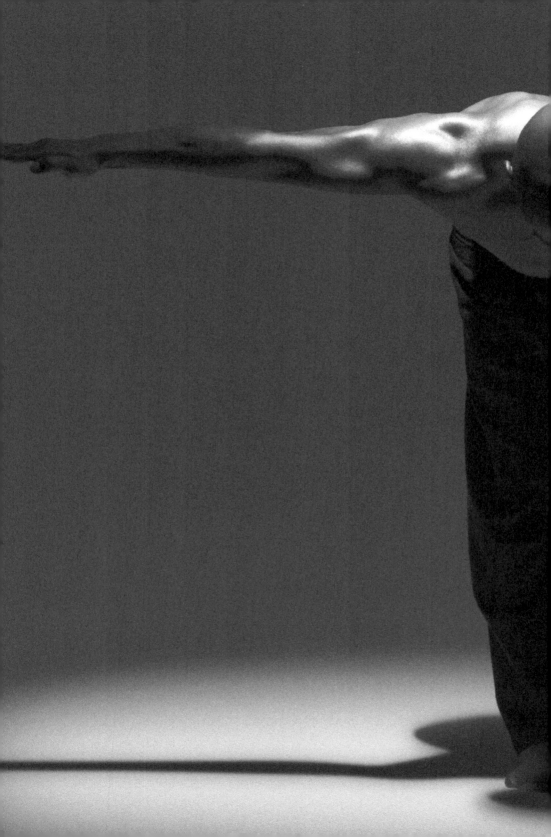

# W·O·L·F

## Wiser Older Leaner Fitter

## WAYNE LÈAL

### with Helen Sutton

Second edition published 2023 by Libri Publishing
First edition published 2019 by Redshank Books

Second edition ISBN 978-1-912969-58-6

First edition ISBN 978-0-9954834-9-1

A CIP catalogue record for this book is available from The British Library

Images courtesy Wayne Lèal

Design by Carnegie Book Production

Libri Publishing
Brunel House
Volunteer Way
Faringdon
Oxfordshire
SN7 7YR

Tel: +44 (0)845 873 3837

www.libripublishing.co.uk

This book is dedicated to my sons Asa, JJ and Leo: be happy.

# PICTURE CREDITS

Wayne Lèal: Pages 10, 12,

Tony Harris: Front and Back Cover, Foreword, Pages 1, 15, 16, 19, 20, 23, 32, 71, 75, 109, 134, 139, 140

Jonathan Knowles: Inside front page 26, 30, 31

Paul Stainthorpe: Pages 40, 47, 110

Victor Frankowski: Pages 46, 51, 54, 66

Richard Pelham: Pages 61

Shutter Stock: Pages 80, 84, 87

Richard Pohle: Page 90

David Bebber: Page 105,

Adobe Stock: Pages 102–3

Champneys own: Page 114

Cat Kennedy: Pages 115, 123, 127, 130, 133

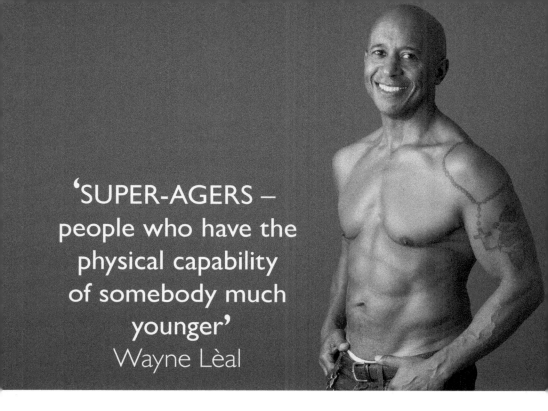

'SUPER-AGERS –
people who have the
physical capability
of somebody much
younger'
Wayne Lèal

# FOREWORD

FACEBOOK, INSTAGRAM, MANY magazines and books describe the keys to a 'better you', with endless motivational or inspirational quotes. Yet people still fail to achieve their goal. This can often be attributed to their inability to value the reciprocal relationship between body and mind.

Your physical self, influences your mind and emotions. Many men want to lose weight, get 'ripped' and gain muscle. They believe that they would have better 'body confidence' if they could achieve this. Women are more complex in many ways, but those who exercise find they are better able to accept, appreciate, and respect themselves – achieving 'body confidence'. Conversely, SUPER-AGERS set a behavioural expectation through regular exercise so that gaining 'body confidence' does not require much effort at all.

As a behavioural change interventionist (Health Coach) my role is to help people develop strategies for positive outcomes – improving their health, exercise, eating, and emotional wellbeing. Basically, I take the unhealthy 'you' from wanting to do something to actually getting it done.

If you go to gym classes, you will see that humans and wolves are really not so very different. In the gym there is a pack mentality, with the gym trainer as the leader. This is in stark contrast to a herd mentality, where individuals act collectively, but without any centralised direction. I am a leader and a 'lone wolf', with my individual training style that is now globally recognised and endorsed by the stringent Yoga Alliance Professionals. This is my Lone W•O•L•F (Wiser Older Leaner Fitter) story, that of a journey along a road less travelled. If you are reading this book, then you were meant to share this part of my life: becoming a Super-Ager.

For years I was caught between two places: who I was perceived to be and who I really am. The truth is that I never fitted neatly into any one category. My achievements serve to show that I rose above the inequality that exists, never accepting that my origins would predetermine my destiny. My experiences along the way, good and bad, forced me to understand and accept life from different people's viewpoints in a myriad of places – though these views were not always in harmony with my own. The most important lesson I have learned is that if you want something to be different in your life then you must do something about it, because it won't change itself.

Art and exercise are the foundation of everything that I do and have always been the main drivers of my life. I have determined the visions of a company's fortunes as a Creative Director, and helped people to transform their minds and bodies as a Health Coach. Art is the ultimate expression of human endeavour – mindful movement, form, shape, imagination, composition, and emotional expression. A body in balance inspires 'confidence', that intangible thing that makes the incredible difference between feeling weak and being powerful.

My training methodology is varied, always changing and adapting, challenging the mind as much as the body. It has evolved as a consequence of my overcoming injuries to every major joint in my body through contact sports and motorcycle accidents. Initially, I had to exercise to stay mobile; now the act of exercising is an integral part of who I am and what I do. My journey has taken many twists and turns, leading me to an unshakeable conviction that my body contributes far more than just physical attributes – it plays a major role in my emotions, learning and relationships, and has taught me the value of using exercise and mindfulness to combat age-related changes.

Ageing is a natural process and is inevitable, but how we age is different for everyone. Lack of fitness in middle age increases your risk of dying so much that it is second only to smoking as a cause of early death. Poor levels of fitness and health awareness contribute to obesity, hypertension, diabetes, and depression.

I am a staunch advocate of the martial arts, boxing, and yoga disciplines because of their united approach to mindfulness and movement. All three emphasise self-control through breath awareness, rather than pure physical force. This is in stark contrast to many popular fitness activities that have an aggressive approach, often leading to muscle strain, joint pain, and ligament tears. Such injuries can, in turn, cause emotional distress, depression, and anxiety; all of which are primary triggers for weight gain and ageing – the very things we are battling against when we exercise! Breath awareness is a fundamental component of my unique SUPER-AGER fitness programme. Mental performance and agility can be considerably improved by increasing oxygen intake. It is said that 9 out of 10 people breathe incorrectly from their chest (shallow breathing or chest breathing) instead of from their abdominal area, causing them to take in less oxygen, thus greatly affecting the quality of their performance and confidence.

During my visits to the Amazon basin in South America, I was privileged to be able to spend time with the indigenous people. They have to move to survive: hunting, farming, fishing and playing rather than consciously exercising. They don't eat processed foods and are largely free from common westernised diseases such as heart disease, cancer, and diabetes. The contrast with my current home, London, is stark. Here I am accustomed to all the modern conveniences of first world living: fast food, modern technology, travel facilities, hospitals and health clubs. The irony is that when I look around, I also see the highest incidences of health problems in the history of mankind.

As a guest speaker, I don't tell people what they need to do, or what they should do. I give them examples of my own personal experiences, ones that others have benefited from, and that they might consider, and relate to.

It's at my SUPER-AGER fitness retreats where the real magic begins to happen; helping you to change your body and give you the mindset for a successful life-fitness outcome.

You can only know something when you have practised every part over and over again. My retreat is the perfect place to do this; enhancing your body awareness, understanding, experiences, and your physical, emotional and spiritual wellbeing. Each day you physically build upon the previous day so that you are giving yourself time to meet your mental, weight and fitness goals; to build focus, strength, endurance, and flexibility.

Having an openness to new experiences will give you a better chance of a successful change, I firmly believe that being fit and healthy is a social responsibility for all of us. You cannot download a new body (yet!), so make the most of the one you've got. By starting to read this book you have taken the first step towards that goal – making the very most of your body. Read on to find out more about how to eat well, how to exercise better, and the benefits of a holistic approach to fitness. It will change your life…

# CONTENTS

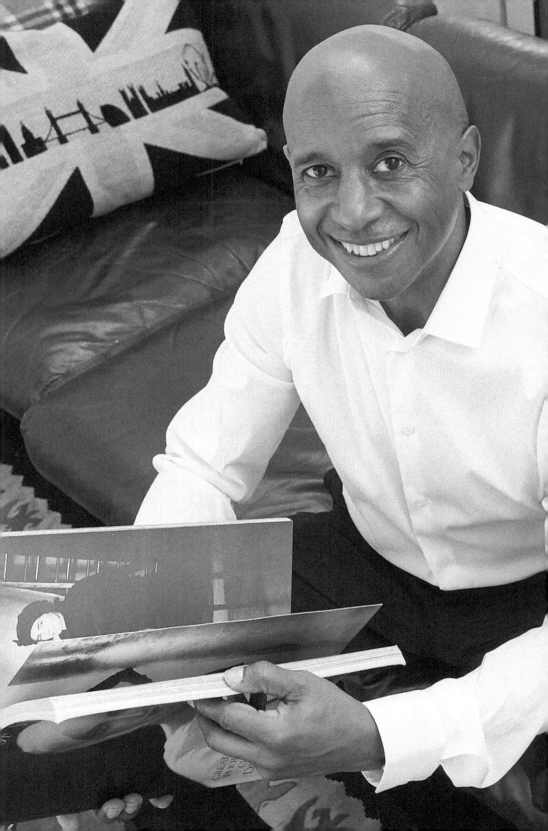

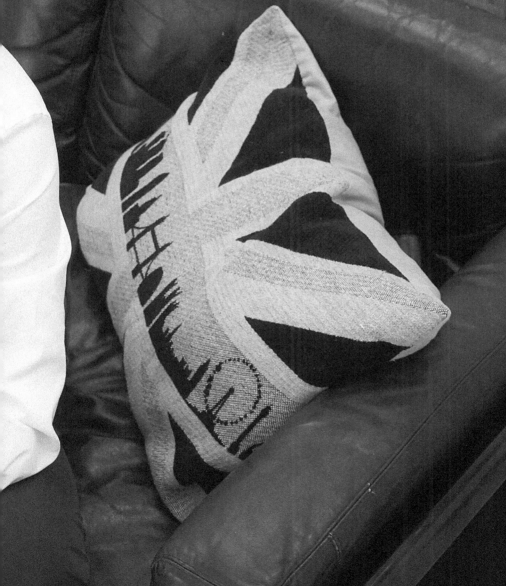

# WHO IS WAYNE LÈAL?

# THE LONE WOLF: WHERE HE CAME FROM, WHERE HE'S BEEN AND WHERE HE'S GOING

GROWING UP, BECOMING the person you want to be for the rest of your life, is a long and complicated process. You can make alterations along the way: change how you look, change your opinions, educate yourself… but a large part of your personality is shaped in early childhood without you even knowing it. The rest is basically sculpting! Some aspects are down to chance and others require willpower and confidence: adding information, chipping off undesirable bits, toning the body and mind a little more with each significant life experience.

Wayne's experiences took him from humble beginnings to where he is now – a roundabout route to his present position as Health Coach, Motivational Speaker and creator of his unique training programme: Super-Ager.

It is said that 'Life is 10% what happens and 90% your response to it'. In a nutshell, Wayne has been through near-death experiences and life's most stressful events and has come out the other side immeasurably stronger and wiser. His response to it all has made him so much more than 'just' a teacher or a speaker – he can empathise with many of his clients, relating to their own experiences that stand in the way of them achieving life goals, and encouraging them to find a way around. He can motivate sportsmen, individuals and captains of industry to set and achieve ambitious goals – because he has 'been there and done that' before them.

The careers master at Chelsea Boys School asked Wayne, then aged 15, what he wanted to be when he left school. He had an eye for the artistic and loved photography, liked the idea of the armed forces but didn't want to fight: 'I want to be an aerial photographer for the RAF,' he said. Such a specific answer floored the careers master just a little – he was used to turning out butchers and carpenters, working-class boys going into working-class jobs. 'How about a car mechanic?' came the hesitant reply, 'You guys are usually quite good at that.'

## Wayne Lèal didn't become a car mechanic…

Born in London, he was malnourished and frail as a child because his mother didn't have enough money to feed herself properly whilst pregnant. Nevertheless, his upbringing was a very disciplined one. His mother's determination to survive and care for her pack made her a figure to whom he owes much of the self-belief that has taken him so far. The closest he had to a father was his older brother, Lincoln, who had come over with his mother from Trinidad in 1956. Between them, they instilled strong values in Wayne and taught him to stand up for himself, no matter what… They lived in south-west London, in an area rife at that time with racial tension, where men called their dogs 'Nigger' – just to be able to shout the name, then laugh and jeer at the likes of Wayne: 'No, not you – the dog!'

He was sent on holidays for deprived children to give his mother a break – Wayne never thought of himself as deprived, but by then she was bringing up his younger brother Paul as well, as a single mother. In these, supposedly fun, holiday camps he would get beaten because of his colour and often wondered what he was doing there.

He was taught to defend himself though – not run away. After being chased home one day, he found that home was not the safe haven he imagined: his mother and brother sent him back out to face his tormentors. It was a hard lesson to learn, but since then he has always faced trouble head on and taken no as feedback, not failure – a challenge rather than a refusal.

At the age of 14, on his way home from school, two white men racially attacked him in broad daylight outside a busy office complex. He was hospitalised; unconscious with a fractured skull and beaten body. He said; 'Afterward, people expected me to hate white people, but I didn't. It just opened a little black boy's eyes to the reality of living in a racist society, through no fault of his own.' From those sorts of beginnings, you either sink or swim. Wayne, of course, swam.

He recalled seeing an ad for a Saturday sales assistant in Jaeger (then one of London's leading fashion stores). A phone call secured him an interview – but of course, nothing had given away his skin colour. Unsurprisingly for the era, he was rejected on arrival at the interview. He told himself, that after this nothing would hold him back, especially not the colour of his skin. The rejection served to increase his resolve though and, just a short while after, he secured an even better job in a men's boutique clothing store called Jones on the Kings Road in Chelsea. Back then Jones was the place to shop; a convergence of London's hippest fashionistas. Wayne befriended the likes of British fashion designer Sir Paul Smith and the late Joseph Ettedgui, who established the fashion brand Joseph. It seemed that the knocks that would have shaken most people's confidence only served to make him stronger.

Lincoln, his late older brother, was involved in the martial arts and the publishing of martial arts books. Wayne also followed his steps into the martial arts and occasionally skimmed through the books wanting to emulate his brother. In one of them, he found the quote that was to become his motto. Everyone needs a 'trigger'; something that resonates with them, summing up where they are going, or helping to push them on when times are hard. He copied the phrase from the book, and tucked it behind a framed painting on the living room wall, to be sure he would never forget. It has been Wayne's 'trigger' for all his life choices and challenging situations:

*To ask may be but a moment of shame, not to ask and remain ignorant is a lifelong shame.*

Following Lincoln's death and after some grieving and painful life experiences, Wayne went to see a faith healer – she told him that each person chooses their family, and he had chosen not to have a father, in order to become his own person. 'A father influences his children: what he did or didn't do in his life, but you have chosen to create yourself – who you are, what you are and where you are going.'

He loved and worshipped his older brother, but Wayne followed an alternative, perhaps more determined, path – albeit always with his brother's and mother's support.

Wayne has always been the firebrand of the family, very different from the others. Lincoln had a Martin Luther King attitude of 'turn the other cheek', whereas Wayne was more the defiant Malcolm X type: '…if someone puts his hand on you, send him to the cemetery.' In essence, these are two different sides of the same coin – each time that a challenge presents itself to us, we have a choice which path we follow.

Back at school, though – Chelsea Boys' School – Wayne was learning one of his most important lessons – to believe in himself. He can still hear his form teacher bellowing to the class, 'It's all about attitude'. True words back then and even more so now. He would walk home through Chelsea, past luxurious houses and fashionable shops and, like a poor boy in a Dickensian story, sneak a look into other people's worlds – planning a different future for himself. Wayne knew that the school didn't expect amazing things of its pupils, so he set himself a personal challenge – to broaden his vocabulary and, with a dictionary at his side, he occasionally read the broadsheet newspapers. He picked them because, as a paperboy, he knew they were the newspapers of choice for the owners of those expensive houses in Kensington & Chelsea. Reading those newspapers didn't contribute to grades or exam results, but he looked up words, widened his vocabulary and educated himself, for himself. These days he doesn't only read the news in the more serious newspapers but has also made the news, having been featured in *The Times*, *The Telegraph* and *The Guardian*. He has also had what he described as a nerve-racking experience: an appearance on BBC news.

At his mother's insistence, Wayne remained in school – she didn't want to see him working in an office, a shop or as a car mechanic. For Wayne, staying on at school bought him more thinking time to figure out what he really wanted to do.

Art and photography were his passion and he cared for little else. Art was also the one subject he did excel at, but with a cruel twist, he was expelled from his Art exam for talking. The tutor who did this had never liked Wayne, and had written in his end of term report: 'Wayne Lèal is the most arrogant pupil I have ever taught.' Wayne remembers looking up the word 'arrogant' and saying to himself: 'No I'm not, I'm confident'.

Prior to his exams, trying to figure out his next step after school, he looked into further education courses and saw the opportunity to apply for a typography course at Camberwell School of Art. Doubting he would get the official entry qualifications, he nevertheless had the confidence to apply – just to see how far he could get. He put together an art portfolio that included classmates' paintings and drawings as well as his own! He did get the interview and was accepted.

He left Camberwell (with a Distinction) and with his first interview was offered a job in advertising. A couple of years later, fancying himself as trendy and something of a 'fashionista', Wayne's eye was caught by an advertisement for a vacancy at *Vogue* magazine. Here again, the race issue reared its ugly head. He was called for an interview, but it actually took place in the reception area rather than an office. The then Art Director spent more time talking to people walking past than interviewing Wayne, and barely glanced at his portfolio. It was evident that for her, his face didn't fit, regardless of his creative ability. At the time he was dating a girl who worked at Mitchell Beazley Publishers. She also wanted to work for *Vogue* but sadly her portfolio was limited because books are developed at a slower pace. Wayne mixed his work in with hers to bulk it up and persuaded her to apply (he has always been very persuasive, with something of a gift for coercing people into doing what he thinks they should rather than what they think they want). She worked at *Vogue* for the next five years…

For Wayne, he had the satisfaction of knowing that his work was good enough to get the job and the only reason it was not going to happen was simply that his face didn't fit. 'At the time I hated the way I was treated but when you've been stripped bare so many times you learn to come back even stronger.'

In 1982 he joined Orbis Publishing as a Design Assistant. Seeing his name in print, on the inside cover of a magazine, was an incredible moment – and the first step in the creation of his own legacy. He became a very competent designer and then Art Editor, leading a small team of designers, but knew that there was more to come.

Several years later a man called Bill Warburton became the new Chairman: a straight-talking, no-nonsense man; there to bring about a change to the company's fortunes. He made several redundancies and brought in his own philosophy, work ethic, and several new ideas. With his wolf-like mentality this was the opening Wayne needed to become the leader of the pack, so he set up a meeting with him and stated: 'We don't have any leadership for the creative look of the company – I want to be the Art Director.' Bill looked at Wayne over his spectacles, without blinking; and explained that it didn't work like that: 'You have to earn a title or a position. First, you earn respect – from me and your colleagues – and then we'll talk.'

Wayne took this on board as an important lesson in life – 'Don't do as I say, do as I do'. So for the coming months he assumed the role, worked very hard and six months later surpassed expectations and was offered the position not just of Art Director but of Creative Director. This was one of the first examples of his hunger to lead by aiming for a specific goal and achieving it – know what you want, say it out loud, commit to it and go for it…

The same counts today with his training programme – an important factor in success is setting a disciplined strategy to achieve the goal. 'Rewire your own thoughts and beliefs about yourself: are you a leader or follower?'

A period followed of representing Orbis Publishing (as part of the Italian de Agostini group) and flying to New York, Germany and, of course, the headquarters in Italy. It was, he admits, a remarkable time in his life. He felt like a real-life executive; jet-setting around the world and staying in the best hotels – and the experience implanted very clearly in Wayne's mind the goal of 'success' in every endeavour.

Being the Creative Director meant Wayne had involvement at several focus groups as part of market research behind style and content of proposed and developing publications. He saw, (as an outside observer at the sessions) how people sat, looked and spoke – and in particular how their body language did not always match their words. It gave valuable insights into the psyche of people in general – invaluable in future years and today as an inspirational speaker – gauging the audiences' reactions, and empathising with them.

As Creative Director, he had teams of designers on different publications, and here he admits to a little quirkiness! In today's world, Personnel and Public Relations would be 'down on him like a ton of bricks', but back then he was fascinated by Linda Goodman's book on star signs, and quietly employed staff using his own personal criteria: keeping fellow water signs in the positions closest to him and basing final interview decisions as much on how people looked as how their portfolio measured up. Here there is definitely a little logic (but apparently a lot of people didn't apply it); at a job interview, how you look is a fair indication of how seriously you take the whole business. As a designer and in publishing, appearance is important – so if a lady arrives at an interview with peeling nail varnish, or a man with scuffed shoes, it may well reflect how observant they will be of the small, but oh so important, details in the world of typography, layouts and visual content.

We like to pretend that what is really important is what is inside a person, but first appearances do count for a lot. As much as anything, how you present yourself reflects your own sense of self-worth. As a young child, Wayne's mother would scrub his one white shirt, drying it in newspaper in the oven if necessary, so that he always went to school looking clean and smart.

After Orbis, in the 1990s, he had the idea of publishing a men's magazine. This was his first experience of using his own money (including remortgaging his home) along with involvement with venture capitalists Stoy Haywood, who had launched a magazine for Classic FM and thought his idea for a men's magazine was fantastic.

A number of others were more cynical, doubting the existence of a marketplace for a men's magazine. Now there are a large number of such publications – back then, however, it was an idea too soon – which meant it might just as well not have been an idea at all. Wayne retreated for a while from the financial loss of independent investment – the wounded wolf needed to lick his wounds.

Working for someone else was a safer option and there followed a stint at *The Mail on Sunday* newspaper. It was one of the best-paid jobs he ever had, with excellent perks and good holidays, but sometimes there is more to life than that. He decreed the job could be done by a 'trained monkey' and cites one of his co-workers as an example of how he so emphatically did not wish to be. The colleague in question, ten years older than Wayne, travelled each day to work wearing a shirt and tie (taken off on arrival at work) carrying a snazzy briefcase, that held nothing more than his sandwiches for lunch. Wayne knew this approach was not for him.

In 1993, his brother Lincoln suddenly died in his sleep. Wayne's world stood still for a while, before spiralling giddily downwards. The next year of his life was a grieving blur; an indiscriminate dabbling in class 'A' drugs and venturing into different religions, looking for a sense of purpose, a reason for who he was, what he was and where was he going. A year later whilst in the Caribbean, his favourite cousin, Diane, told him he should go to Guyana (the Amazon Basin), and immerse himself in nature for a deep, mental, physical, emotional and spiritual journey.

The trip proved to be an overwhelming experience; especially when he befriended an Amerindian (the indigenous population) called Lincoln and his community. Wayne said, 'I had never met another Lincoln in my life before that day really, what were the chances of that happening?' A few days later he was invited to go night hunting with Lincoln and his

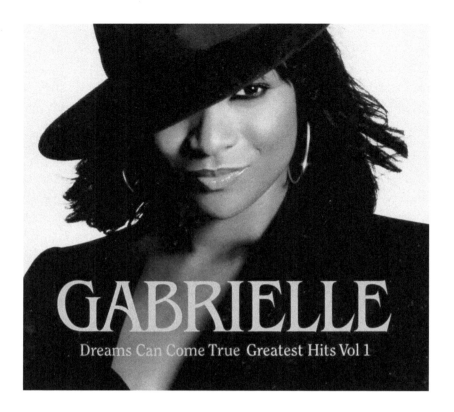

**GABRIELLE**

Dreams Can Come True Greatest Hits Vol 1

friends. It was pitch black, and when he asked where the torches were he was told that they used the moonlight and that his eyes would adjust in a little while. Wayne said; 'For a short while, I was blind, putting all of my trust in Lincoln as I stumbled through the darkness of the rainforest. After repeatedly saying my brother's name, I suddenly felt his presence beside me. At that moment I had an overwhelming feeling to let go of all the emotional turmoil that I had inside following his death. For over a year I had denied my emotions and, as my eyes adjusted to the moonlight, there was also an inner clarity that released me from my self-inflicted prison of loss and pain. In that moment I knew my brother was okay, and it was time for me to go forward and live my life to the fullest. When I left Guyana it was with a new perspective on life, people, actions, and emotions. No longer caught up in 'things' such as job, car, home, clothes, and money.'

On returning home to London, it was the combination of this experience and his family that ultimately brought Wayne back down to earth. He had two sons who needed him as a father, as a role model. He also had his own life on hold, with all the aspirations and possibilities hanging in limbo.

In 1997 he decided to take on the biggest challenge he could think of: to organise a major musical event to raise awareness and funds for the treatment of Sickle Cell Anaemia and Aplastic Anaemia – two blood disorders that affect mostly black and Asian people. He called it 'Gene Aid' and it was showcased at London's Shepherds Bush Empire, featuring Gabrielle, Keith Washington, and Omar. *The Mail on Sunday* (where he worked) was not known for feel-good 'black' stories back then; so when he took his idea to the then Editor, it not surprisingly fell on deaf ears. In stark contrast though, *The Guardian* newspaper took up the story and ran a two-page spread about Sickle Cell and his campaign, Gene Aid. Unbeknown to Gabrielle, she rehearsed her famous hit 'Dreams Can Come True' to an audience of one: Wayne. How fitting, you may think.

Now firmly believing that anything was possible, he forged ahead with the next phase of his career; and took a second stab at publishing his own magazine. He called it *The Public Eye* and it was a news magazine with a mission. It aimed to deliver the news from a black perspective; a minority voice but free from fear, discrimination, prejudice or racism.

Again using his own money he co-published the *The Public Eye*, with an old school friend, who edited whilst Wayne created. They both gained an unparalleled insight into the world of celebrity power and political rivalry.

*The Public Eye* struggled to obtain advertising, though. Wayne said what he was doing gave minorities an educated voice. He felt that black people are most likely to be commented on socially as entertainers, athletes, musicians or criminals but there are very few articles talking about black people in positions of power; company owners or captains of industry. He said black people are primarily consumers; they don't own blue-chip companies, stores or car companies. This made it all the more significant; the importance of publishing *The Public Eye* itself.

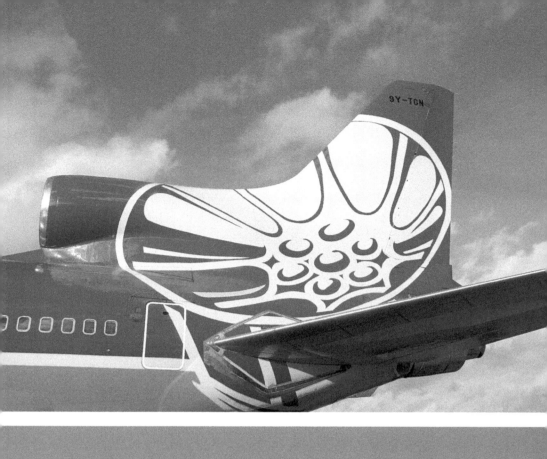

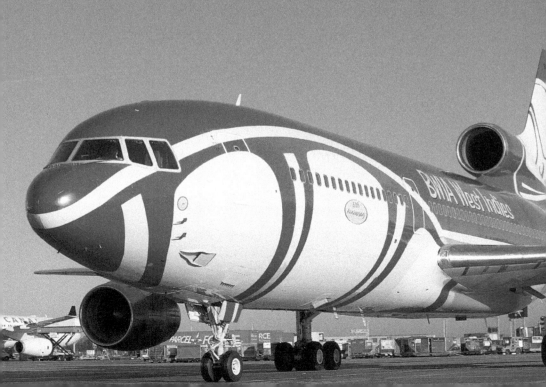

*The Public Eye* was shortlisted as Magazine of the Year, and yet they struggled to obtain advertising – which is, of course, the bloodline and mainstay of any publication. The challenge to survive month to month took its toll – *The Public Eye* eventually folded after 3 years, but was a fantastic journey and a learning experience for Wayne.

Sometimes it's a case of seeing an opportunity and grabbing it with both hands. There are many people who are good at what they do. Some are excellent, and there are those that are unstoppable. This is Wayne, unstoppable in his own world because he doesn't compete with anyone but himself. He says; 'I'm not motivated by money – it's never been about the money. I just enjoy challenging experiences and giving it my all.'

Before and during his time at *The Public Eye*, Wayne designed the livery for British West Indian Airways – which was, for a while, the number one transatlantic airline in the Caribbean.

Wayne's livery design incorporated the Steel Pan; an instrument that was created by the working class man and was representative of their fight against oppression and yearning for a sense of belonging. BWIA's then Chairman Lawrence Duprey said the new livery design 'symbolised Caribbean culture'.

The following was Wayne's design mission statement:

### 'A symbol is the core of a company's identity and philosophy'

And he went on to explain his inspiration for the design; the steel pan being globally recognised as 'Caribbean', how his artwork was emblematic, easily identifiable and memorable, and could be reproduced in many formats.

Wayne saw the Caribbean airline project as the pinnacle of his creative work. The stakeholders were a nation of people, most challenging and most diverse that he had ever experienced. He knew that he needed to create an iconic brand image of the nation and the Steel Pan was the single unifying factor that reflected the core values of the Caribbean people, their diversity, and dynamism. He also had to think about how people in other countries would perceive the brand.

The last hurdle prior to his design being chosen was the large-scale audit that involved public officials, business owners and everyday working man and woman. It was nerve-racking until it was announced that his design had been chosen.

In 2000, Wayne was nominated and won a Small Businessman of the Year Award, for co-publishing *The Public Eye* and for his design of the BWIA airline livery. The award ceremony was held at the prestigious Dorchester Hotel in Hyde Park and Wayne was seated at the front with other nominees, who had all achieved something significant in their respective fields. During the course of the evening, Wayne asked the waiter for a beer, but was informed that he would have to go to the bar at the rear of the ballroom since only champagne and fine wine was served at the table. Wayne duly moved to the bar and sat drinking a bottle of beer. He had come on his motorbike and, reasoning that he wasn't going to win anything and would only be seen from the waist up at the table, was sporting a smart tuxedo, waistcoat, and cravat up above, but leather jeans and biker boots down below. He missed the announcement of his category and missed his own name being called as the winner. The spotlight swung to his empty seat and a former colleague from *The Mail on Sunday* newspaper shouted to him, 'They've called your name, you've won!' Wayne called out 'I'm over here' – and the spotlight swung again. He had no speech planned and made his way, truly nervous, to the stage to collect his award. He mumbled something – to this day he has no idea what – as he raised the award aloft!

We mentioned motorbikes. They have been a huge feature in Wayne's life. As a small boy, he was taken for rides in a sidecar. His mother rode pillion in Trinidad, his older brother owned a Triumph motorbike he had rebuilt.

Wayne, who owns a motorbike to this day, deems riding one the closest you can come to absolute Zen – having discovered to his own detriment

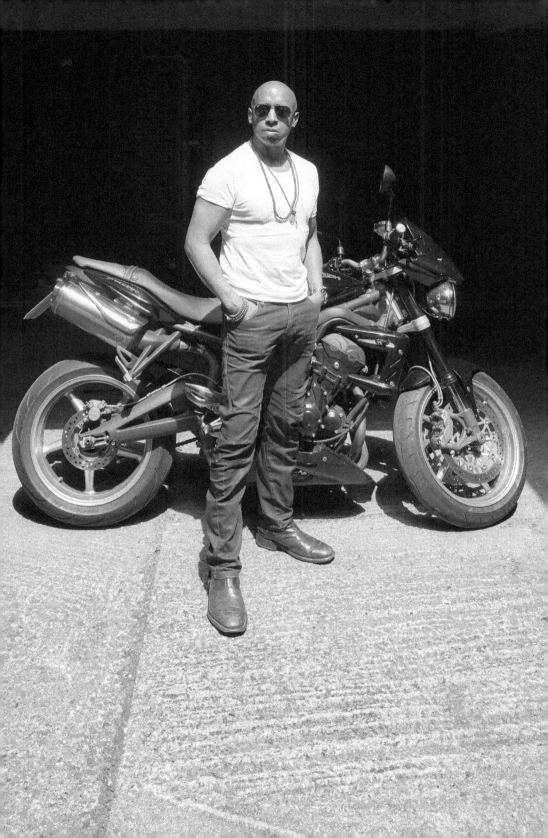

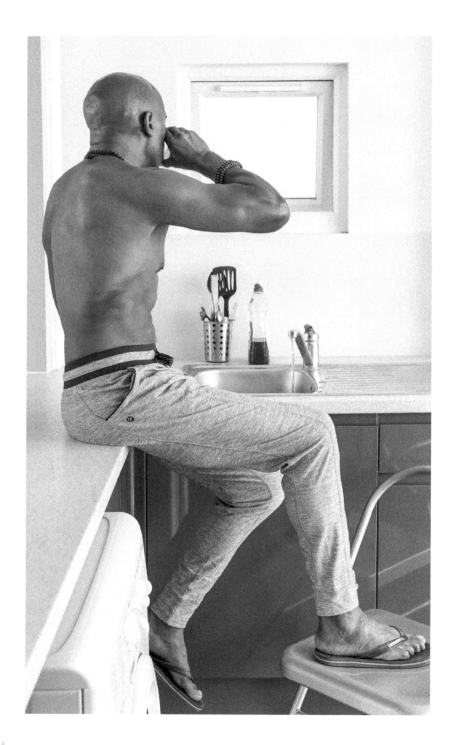

that the consequences of not being completely 'in the moment' on a bike can be pretty dire.

One accident saw him and his younger brother (Paul) riding together on the Continent, and his brother careering into the back of Wayne's Triumph motorbike at 60mph; writing off his own Moto-Guzzi motorbike and being flown back to the UK by air ambulance.

The most vivid and near-death motorbike experience though was around fifteen years ago. Wayne was on his way to train young boxers at the All Stars Boxing Club when a minicab driver in front of him executed an illegal U-turn. Wayne slammed into the side of the car. He and his motorbike flipped over the bonnet and he saw, as if in slow motion, the driver's face behind the windscreen and the silhouette of his 1200cc Buell motorbike in the sky above his head.

He came round later with a paramedic shining a light into his eyes. He was numb from the waist down – the handlebar of his bike had speared his groin, and that would later result in him needing a hip operation. Several months later he received a letter informing him that the driver was being prosecuted, so he attended court. Entering the witness room, he was taken aback to see a number of people and asked them if they were there for the bike accident case. The full impact of the event only really hit him when he thanked them for turning up and they all looked incredulously at him. They had felt compelled to come as witnesses to the accident because they were all sure that he had died.

He has also, at various points in time, dislocated both of his shoulders, had four major knee operations, a bone graft in his jaw, a hip resurface and been stabbed in the eye with a fork (actually by his cousin and not a racial attack – the fork was flicked at him in play but, with greasy fingers, it slipped. Moorfield's checked him out and his eye survived!), broken his nose boxing, burst a vein in his shoulder when injured in a dooring incident and survived a meaningless attack by a gang of seven men who were charged for the offence.

Having worked his way up in publishing, graphics, and magazines, Wayne gradually became a little disillusioned with the creative world. Nobody had an opinion at the inception of a project but once a design was presented everyone became an expert critic. He realised that creativity is so subjective and everything so open to opinion. He was in need of something that was clearly either right or wrong, that fitted or didn't; without discussion and regardless of opinion.

So he did a plumbing course! His friends were somewhat shocked, but he logically pointed out to them that, as a form of livelihood, it more or less guaranteed income since 'no-one likes to touch their own s\*\*\*, let alone someone else's! So where there's s\*\*\*, there's money!' His brother Paul gave up his job at an architectural firm to join him; Paul achieved the highest mark in a City & Guilds plumbing course – apparently being a genius for the small details.

They teamed up together and started a company. They soon moved from general repairs to employing a team of ten men to work for them doing extensive house refurbishments, thus adding creativity back into the mix!

Prior to this more practical career strand, Wayne studied NLP, Neuro-Linguistic Programming, which uses patterns of how we think and communicate to help modify or alter behaviour. In 2003 he developed his own variation on the theory: Neuro Physical Training, which related more closely to links between movement (i.e. exercise) and emotion. This was pioneered in a London Primary School with considerable success for the children and teachers concerned, but funding issues prevented it from spreading further afield.

The most notable achievement during his building career was, in Wayne's eyes, the purchase of a building in Fulham, which they gutted and rebuilt to their own specifications. A part of it is now Wayne's home and another section his fitness studio. He said, 'Nothing beats building your own home'. Plenty of people have homes built to their own

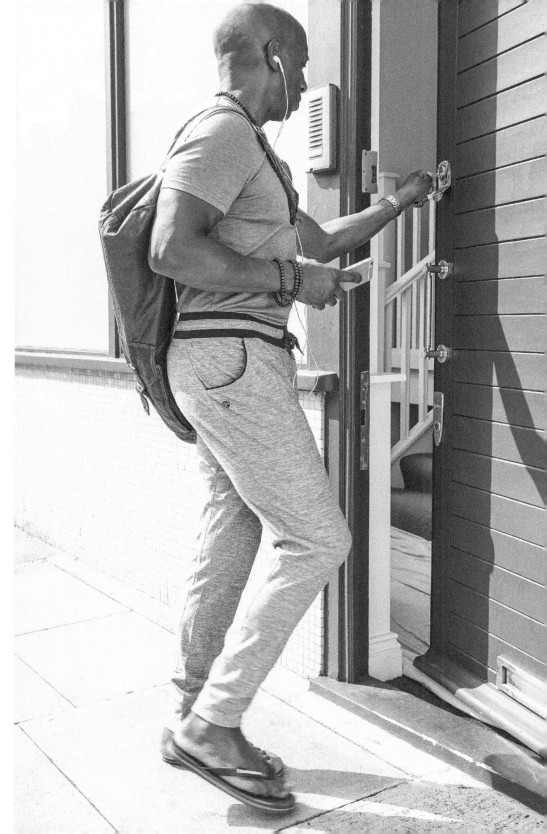

requirements, but not many have the patience, tenacity, resourcefulness and the ultimate sense of achievement of having done it themselves!

Inevitably, all good things come to an end – or rather recessions return. There were a number of large projects pending, but overheads were equally large and, when promised work didn't materialise, a decision had to be made.

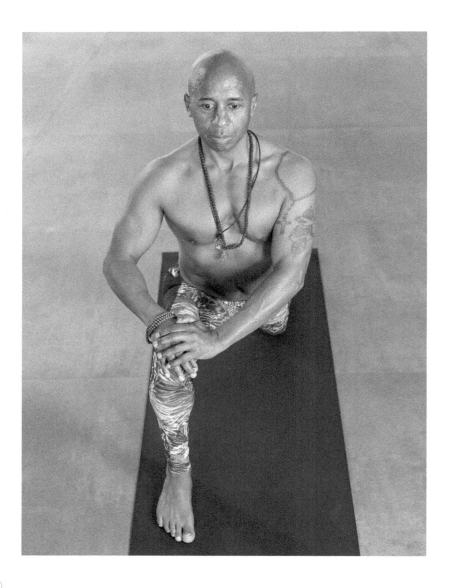

## Where to now? What goal to set for himself next?

He had built his own fitness studio in the building that also contains his apartment. Being aware of his body, fitness had always been a vocation. He'd studied Martial Arts alongside his big brother, dabbled in boxing, taught fitness classes, and practiced yoga.

He had learned so many life lessons, overcome so many injuries and learned about his body in the process. His late mother once remarked: 'You've spent more time in the hospital than you have on holidays'. Art and Wellbeing were interwoven into his life as a social activity; a means of rehabilitation after injury and a lifeline when the world seemed a little out of sync.

He actually taught his first fitness class over 35 years ago and continued to occasionally teach part-time throughout his life. Now he combined his years of experience in the field of training and fitness, with his creative mind and passion for life, in a quest to find a way to exercise that could work at every level and every age to bring out the best. The path was a clear one and Wayne turned down it: away from construction and graphic design into fitness, away from creativity with words and images and into creativity with the mind and body.

As part of his passion for self-improvement over the years he amassed a whole array of qualifications as well as personal experience (since paper proof of your ability does matter too!) He is a Senior Yoga Teacher, a qualified Personal Trainer, an ABAE Assistant Boxing Coach and a Master NLP Practitioner. He also studied hypnotherapy and the whys and wherefores around the science of fitness; and his own physical injuries led him to search for realistic exercise solutions.

He was fascinated by theoretical models explaining processes of changing apparently ingrained behaviour and ultimately based his very own exercise programme on the precepts of the Transtheoretical Model of Behavioural Change.

Yoga melded with other low impact but high effect exercises – water resistance exercises and rebounding – to form two interchangeable mind and body exercise programmes that offer people the choice. According to Wayne, both men and women tend to do the same exercise as they were doing in their early years, simply because it's what they know or have seen others doing. But it is not necessarily right for their bodies that have reached their physical peak. This can cause them to become more injury prone, lose muscle mass and, for the average person, to get heavier at the same time.

His training has worked for men and women looking to regain control of their bodies after a few years of neglect; for young and aspirational gym goers looking for an alternative, lower impact form of exercise; for captains of industry keeping themselves fit and healthy as well as their businesses; and for sportsmen looking for that extra edge to get them over that last hurdle and to their ultimate goal.

Wayne's physical statistics are pretty good too; with minimal body fat (12%) and optimum muscle mass, proving that fitness can be a broader notion than simply an hour in the gym. Linking his programme to individual realistic goals, to mindfulness and to a view of living a longer healthier life rather than 'just' a toned figure, he has turned fitness into a lifestyle.

### Wayne's training started in his studio, but spread…

He runs Teacher Training courses and gives workshops in resorts as far afield as Thailand, where he says: 'Encountering different nationalities and social groups makes me more creative and sometimes has me questioning my own reality – but it also made me realise that people are basically the same the world over. Those who have or can find a sense of inner self-worth are those with the confidence to achieve and succeed'.

He has at times lived a five-star lifestyle and been invited to dinner by billionaires, causing him sometimes to pinch himself as he marvels that he is essentially an average guy, made good. He laughingly says; 'A

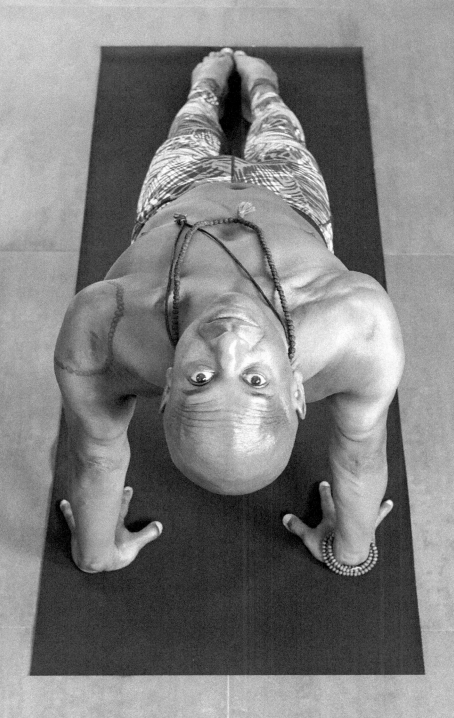

round of drinks for them, could buy my food shopping for a month', and yet people with the most enviable wealthy lifestyles ask him for advice not only on health and fitness, but how to live their lives – placing responsibility for their whole wellbeing in Wayne's hands.

After giving a yoga class in 'The Yoga Barn' in Bali, he was invited to attend a group philosophy meeting of spiritually minded souls. He listened to them politely but felt somewhat out of place: they were intensely discussing finding themselves – and all Wayne could think of was how he had spent his life so far creating himself.

Mindfulness does play a vital role in his life and his training of others, though. The ability to be intensely aware of yourself, to the extent of detachment from current situations and visualisation of others was a key in his training of certain athletes and can work for all of us to instil discipline, confidence and focus at times when we are more inclined towards panic.

Closer to home, he has been a regular motivational speaker at Champneys – the quintessentially English health spa – giving talks and workshops on exercise and mindfulness to combat age-related changes.

Is he good at what he does? Billionaires and world-class athletes ask him for advice on how to live their lives…

We all know a person like Wayne, whose mere presence can silence a crowded room. How did he get there, though? How has he achieved that level of confidence in himself?

Some people have that 'je ne sais quoi'; the self-assurance that gives them an ability to lead, convince and influence others. Wayne's eldest son puts out his cigarette in response to a glance from his father across a crowded bar. He commands respect over love from his 'children' (two are grown men, but still his sons!), but I suspect that deep down they love him more because of it. He now has two grandchildren as well, though, which may prove the first instance of them twisting Wayne round their little fingers… a taste of his own medicine!

No one event has decisively shaped Wayne's life, yet the twists and turns on his initial career path were always held together by the thread of art and fitness. We are all a collage of the events that happen and the parts that we play along the way.

Wayne at times has the characteristics of a 'Lone Wolf' with his individual take on life, and it's not easy to stay that original in a world where everyone is constantly trying to fit in – where being part of a group is the place to be. Wayne speaks of an occasion when he was meeting up with some friends. He arrived early at Piccadilly Circus – a corner of London that he hadn't visited in quite some time. He sat at an outdoor café, watching the hustle and bustle of the world passing by but separated from it all. He was mindful and yet a person apart; aware of being just a speck in the universe, temporarily unaffected by the world around him. Being happy with only yourself for company takes practice and self-assurance!

Wayne has learned from experience, and others, in turn, are learning from him; that everyone needs a realistic goals in life. Goals that can be achieved with determination and self-belief. He says 'Life changes are made one step at a time, but you will cover an incredible distance in good health if you can just keep moving…'

There are many people who are good at what they do. Some are excellent, and there are those that are unstoppable. This is Lèal, unstoppable because he doesn't compete with anyone but himself. He says, 'S••t happens, but you must believe there are no limits, because everything is possible.' It is that unrelenting drive and positivity of thought that make him an exceptional and inspirational Health Coach.

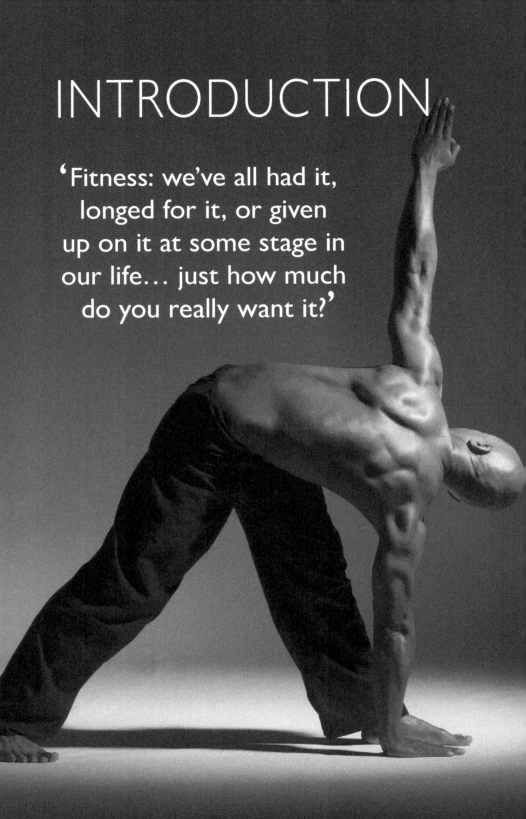

# INTRODUCTION

'Fitness: we've all had it, longed for it, or given up on it at some stage in our life… just how much do you really want it?'

# CHANGE YOUR LIFESTYLE – CHANGE YOURSELF

EXERCISE FADS AND fashions come and go over the years – some founded on common sense, others less so; and some with slightly bizarre roots.

The treadmill, now a standard fixture in every gym, was once a punishment device in prisons! Designed by Sir William Cubitt in 1818 and called a Treadwheel, it was used as a form of hard labour for prisoners in at least 44 prisons across the UK. As men walked the 'endless staircase', the big wheel turned, and gears pumped water or crushed grain (so not just punished but exploited). Even Oscar Wilde was compelled to spend time on it whilst doing time for indecency. At a prison just outside New York, men spent up to 10 hours a day on the treadwheel. Ultimately, though, it was deemed too cruel, and abolished. A little later, in 1913, the first patent was filed for a treadmill; an update on the same idea, and nowadays gym goers worldwide voluntarily subject themselves to 'punishment' in the search for fitness!

Fitness, however, is not just the rock-hard abs, the bulging muscles, or the tight butt – it is the whole 'feeling good, looking good, being the best, you can' package. A fleeting New Year's resolution is not enough. Fitness needs to be an entire lifestyle choice.

In our era, medical science has come up with ever greater innovations and advances that have pushed up the median age throughout the developed world. Yet we have the highest ever incidences of weight-related diseases. Obesity, stress, ageing: all are major preoccupations in the modern world; not only for ourselves but also for scientists attempting to quantify them, determine why, and ultimately find ways to stop them happening. It is generally agreed that there are ways to slow down ageing, to speed up weight loss, to reduce stress – with the most effective therapy available to everyone being exercise. The challenge is finding the way that best helps you to tackle your specific issues.

In addition to exercise; diet and lifestyle also play crucial roles in how we look and how we feel. Hence these are the areas to alter if we want to see and feel a change in ourselves.

There has been a myriad of scientific studies over the years related to the stages involved in the process of behavioural change, the hurdles to be jumped and the series of activities and emotions to be gone through.

*What if someone took all the studies and every theory related to them and amalgamated them into one global theory of behavioural change?* It's been done! It's called the Transtheoretical Model of Behavioural Change.

*Then what if someone took that model and based an exercise programme on those proven concepts, helping people to change their perceptions and hence themselves, both inside and out?*

It's been done – and it works. Thirty-five years of scientific study into behavioural change and Wayne Lèal's thirty-five years of experience in training, have been combined to develop his **Super-Ager** mind and body programme – to enable each of us to stay fitter longer and to combat age-related changes. And – it will also give us a better understanding of who we are and where we are going, to transform ourselves into the best that we can be.

This book is much more than a fitness guide. It tells the story of Wayne Lèal who has experienced incredible success and bad luck at first hand as a result of being attracted to life at the extreme. He has at some time or another injured virtually every major joint in his body, but through training and determination has emerged stronger. He emphatically proclaims wellbeing as a key element in defining who we are, and over the years has experimented with numerous training disciplines. This exploration has culminated in the creation of Super-Ager Fitness, a life lesson we can all learn.

The WHO (World Health Organisation) defines health as a state of complete physical, mental and social wellbeing – all the same basic characteristics claimed by religion. For years, people who have attended

Wayne's retreats, workshops and talks say that his words are, for them, the definitive 'gospel' on good health. This book aims to spread those words and give everyone who needs it that final push; setting them on a new path to fitness. His training principles will help you set realistic goals for yourself and implement an exercise strategy to achieve them. His programme is backed up by studies and scientific research into behavioural change, acknowledging the factors that affect everyone's level of fitness and wellbeing. It shows how positive yet simple lifestyle changes such as reducing stress and increasing exercise adapted to your body, your age and your level of fitness, can enable you to achieve truly wonderful things – strengthening your mind and body in order to be happy and healthy.

It has been tried and tested by athletes, captains of industry and the man, or woman, in the street. Their stories are told here – how goals ranging from winning a world title to simply walking upstairs unaided can be achieved if you set your mind, and body, to it. If his training programme were packaged as a pharmaceutical drug, it would be a very valuable one!

Super-Ager Fitness, whilst creative and doable, is less about the exercise itself and more about the way it makes you feel, giving you the impetus to transform yourself. Change is a process, not a one-off event – a series of moments and adjustments in your attitude and hence your life. Putting yourself in a positive frame of mind and having a specific goal to focus on helps you to a place where you feel confident with your own self-image; with how others see you on the outside and how you see yourself on the inside.

We all have insecurities, but that shouldn't stop anyone from making the best of who and what they are and what they are trying to achieve. Small changes can have a big effect. Accept that you can advance just one step at a time, as long as you keep moving forward. Once you have identified and accepted that what you want is actually achievable, you set your personal goal, devise a realistic strategy and you are on your way there, to where you want to be; to be the best of you.

For Wayne Lèal, the development of Super-Ager Fitness has been a lifelong journey of learning and discovery; a remarkable story of self-creation, and of his own and others' transformation.

Wayne's career path has taken many turns, but almost every door he's tried has led him to success. Wayne says success is loving what you do. He has worked in publishing, design, building, fitness training, NLP, motivational speaking and wellbeing; setting himself a goal in each instance – and fulfilling it. This book charts his journey and for you, it can be the start of a journey of discovery of your own; a life transition from where you are right now, to where you really want to be.

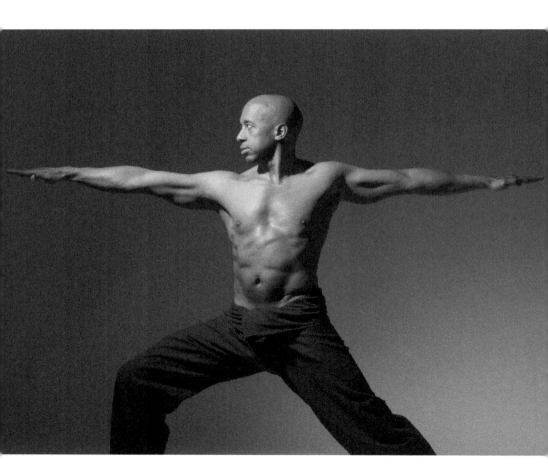

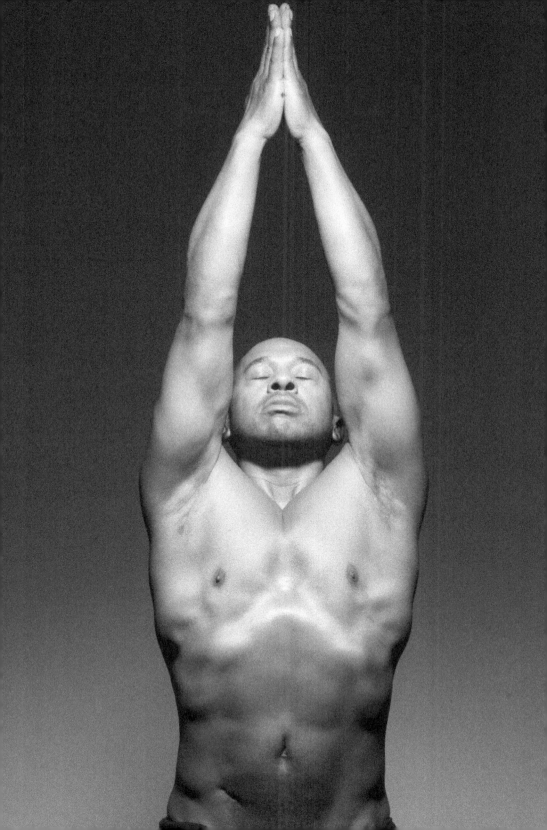

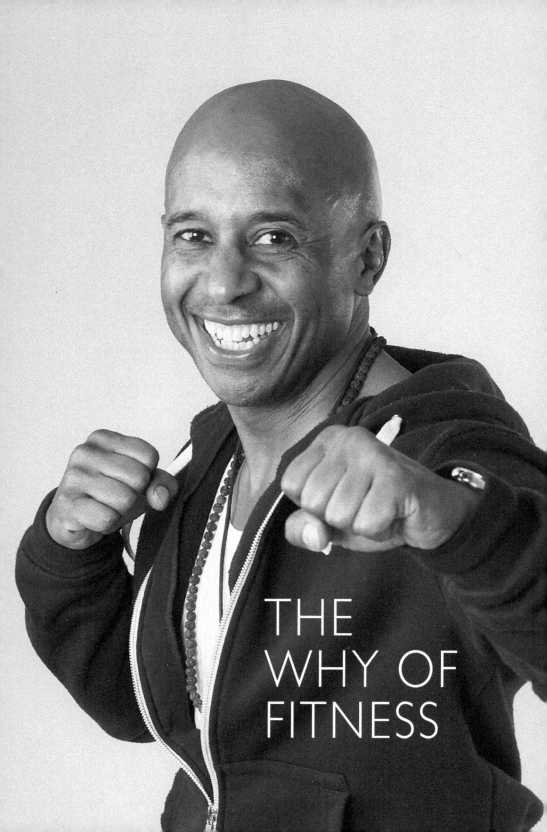

THE
WHY OF
FITNESS

# WHY GET FIT?

NOBODY IS BORN with wisdom. It is something we must discover for ourselves; knowledge from a series of experiences that forms our identity. The discipline to exercise is not necessarily there in people who need to do it the most. When you want to exercise, but don't, it most likely results from not being sufficiently motivated. You will only achieve something if you really want it – it's as simple as that. This is the reason why Super-Ager was created with its mindful approach for a successful life-fitness outcome.

*'It is beyond a doubt that all our knowledge begins with experience'*

Immanuel Kant

The underlying philosophy of Super-Ager Fitness is that real strength begins in the mind. Our physical state directly affects our mental and emotional wellbeing. This is about how we feel, think, behave and communicate. Looking after your body is as important as taking your state of mind.

Most people know, deep down, that they are leading ever more sedentary lives. Yet it's not so easy to change your behaviour. Life has become increasingly automated and we have many labour-saving devices. Laziness tells us to take it easy, to sit back after a hard day at the office, eat that ready meal, and watch that reality show. It takes a lot of discipline, willpower and incentive to change our habits, to get up and get moving. But here are some of the reasons why we should…

## BACK PAIN

The spine reflects the overall health of your body and no matter how fit and athletic you are, a wrong move could injure your lower back. The lower back is subject to injury, twisting, or a sudden movement can cause muscles or ligaments to stretch or develop microscopic tears. Over time, poor posture can also lead to muscle strain or other soft tissue problems.

## STRESS

Our wellbeing can be challenged by work-related stress, which is the second biggest occupational health problem in the UK (after back problems). When people feel under pressure at work, they tend to work harder to try to close the gap between what they are achieving and what they think they should be achieving. Stress can paralyse people's ability to get on with life – it can make them feel that there is no hope, and no point, in carrying on.

## OBESITY

In the UK, 70% of adults are classed as being overweight or obese, costing the UK billions every year – and this figure is continuing to rise. The obesity epidemic now affects nearly every business, country, income level, race, ethnicity and age group, Obesity rates among children have been increasing and become a major concern for parents around the world. An obese woman, compared with a healthy weight woman, is:

- almost thirteen times more likely to develop diabetes

- more than four times more likely to develop high blood pressure

- more than three times more likely to have a heart attack

Scary statistics – and obesity starts young! A recent Health Survey for England found that 31% of children between the ages of two and fifteen are classed as overweight or obese. Television, computers and electronic games are keeping children inside and inactive.

## AGE SLOWS US DOWN TOO...

Getting old is inevitable – the birthdays keep coming even if we stop counting or refuse to blow out the candles on the cake. Looking and feeling old is a little more within our control though...we can't stop the clock, scientists have proven that with the right mental attitude and physical activity; we can slow the aging process down a little.

As you age your muscles get smaller, and as they shrink, the fat around them increases. And we all know that too much fat is not healthy. Weight and stress problems, in general, induce age-related issues to hit earlier.

Cortisol is the chemical produced in our bodies in response to stress and an excessive amount of it weakens muscles and degrades bones, as well as being fat inducing. Hence activity or specific exercise that reduces our stress levels and our weight will, in turn, increase fitness and feelings of wellbeing and counteract to some extent the issues of frailty that come with ageing. Stronger muscles, gained through exercise, will decrease pain and increase control and range of movement.

Some people do naturally seem to age 'better', or at least more slowly, than others – but studies of twins living in contrasting locations have shown that lifestyle accounts for 75% of the influence, leaving just 25% for the genes. A study by the BBC of 55-year-old twins in the USA found that the twin living a relaxed lifestyle in the country, eating healthily and horse riding for exercise, weighed slightly more but was biologically two years younger than her sister who was living a high-powered, more stressful lifestyle in town. Of course, we don't all have the option or the inclination to head off to the country and decline every stressful situation – but we can be aware of what to aim for and what to avoid!

## TELOMERES

We already know that exercise builds strength and endurance, enhances flexibility, lowers blood pressure, helps ward off many diseases, and burns calories to help us maintain a healthy weight. But exercise also has an anti-ageing effect at a cellular level. Tim D. Spector, a professor of genetic epidemiology at King's College in London, led a study on the effects of exercise on ageing. The study found that exercise appears to slow the shrivelling of the protective tips on bundles of genes inside cells (called telomeres), which means a slowing of the whole ageing process. 'These data suggest that the act of exercising may actually protect the body against the aging process,' said Spector.

The benefits of exercise go beyond the physical. Studies show that staying physically fit also keeps your brain healthy into old age – including compelling evidence of a link between aerobic fitness and cognitive preservation. What's good for your heart is good for your head!

Exercise is the most transformative thing you can do for your brain today. A single workout will improve reaction times, and will immediately increase levels of neurotransmitters like dopamine, serotonin, and noradrenaline; these improvements will last for at least two hours. The hippocampus and prefrontal cortex two areas are more susceptible to neurodegenerative diseases and cognitive decline in ageing.

The good news is that the brain is like a muscle, and doing exercise three to four times a week for a minimum 30 minutes each session (including aerobic exercise) will protect your brain and take longer for these diseases to actually have an effect. You will be changing the trajectory of your life for the better.

When it comes to what type of exercise, it doesn't have to be vigorous to have a great effect – a 2014 study by the *European Journal of Preventative Cardiology* found that yoga was just as effective as more rigorous cardiovascular exercise at reducing the risk of heart disease. Not to mention, of course, that, being low impact, it is much kinder to bones and joints which tend to become stiffer with age, and with practice, it will improve the flexibility and strength of those joints!

### *When people start stopping, that's when they start getting old.*

For older people, as with any age group, exercise can have an important social aspect to it too – learning a new skill such as yoga, dancing, tennis, or any exercise conducted in a group setting will stretch you physically through the exercise, mentally through the learning of it and socially through interacting with others in the class – increasing fitness and wellbeing in every area of your life.

Wayne says, 'Everywhere you look there are people doing their best to deny the disappointment that they have in their own bodies'. In his Wellness Talks, Wayne has a way of motivating people who are ordinarily not really an exercise sort of person. As hard as they've tried, they've never liked going to the gym. They may have hired a personal trainer for accountability, but even that was not enough to do regular exercise. He simply reasons that when you first start your fitness programme don't force yourself, just make sure that you stick with it and never quit. Discipline is the only way to get there.

- *Set a goal – and make it one you really want*

- *Develop a strategy toward achieving life-fitness*

- *Increase muscle mass and improve weight loss*

- *Improve your cardio, flexibility, and strength in middle age and beyond*

- *Develop a mindful practice that can alter your biological age.*

Behaviour is achievement oriented, we work towards a specific measurable point – losing x number of kilos or xx number of centimetres off our waistline. Whether you are aiming to run the marathon for the first time, or in your personal best time, or to come first in the parents' race on sports day or 'just' to walk up two flights of stairs without getting out of breath…you have to gear your goal to your personal lifestyle; aiming high, but within the notions of what is possible.

Getting in shape is a different journey depending on where you start from – we are not all out to lose the same amount of weight or reach the same levels of fitness, so it's important that your own goal is realistic for you!

Set a reason – know your 'why', and make it strong, stronger than all the excuses and problems that might challenge it. Better health, better looks, better feelings: all are worthy if you really want them enough to keep you going.

Start – Super-Ager Fitness is simple and doable. There is a general and uncontested conclusion among the scientists that exercising will make you happier and healthier – boosting memory, concentration, and mental sharpness as well as keeping your weight down, your heart healthy and your muscles strong.

Start small but keep going – once you begin, don't stop! It doesn't have to be a lengthy, sweaty exercise session every day: set a small goal of ten minutes of daily JumpGa exercise that has to be completed, and count everything else as an extra achievement. That way you are much more likely to find yourself rewarding the positive rather than feeling ashamed of the negative.

Talking of positive – concentrate on what you have to gain, not what you have to give up! Being fit makes you feel better, look better, and live longer – what is there not to like?

Getting fit, changing yourself, achieving a goal – they are not one-off events, though, they are processes – taking time and commitment. It might sound scary – but if the goal is worth reaching and the process is planned, it can almost be fun, and it is certainly worthwhile.

Wayne believes that it is important to identify what it is that you want first – why you want to change. The most important factor is the desire to change 'something', but you have to also know, more specifically, what you want to achieve: otherwise, how will you know when you get there?

He says; 'Our motivation for exercise changes as we go through life therefore, it's our discipline that will outweigh our motivation'.

The young among us are concerned with body image. There are issues of vanity, competition or peer pressure; the need to look the best you can.

### Midlife is the end of the beginning.

Those further into adulthood are motivated to exercise by the need to maintain health and image, to ward off illness, or fight the odd extra kilo.

Once past middle age, 'older' people tend to turn to exercise to rejuvenate themselves, to prolong life and help with mobility issues.

Whatever it is that prompts us, Wayne says; 'It's essential to remember that we see discipline as a muscle that you can train to improve and make stronger'. So it goes without question that you will soon form a habit with small acts of self-control that will make your discipline stronger and more determined to achieve your goal and to preserve your youth right down to your DNA.

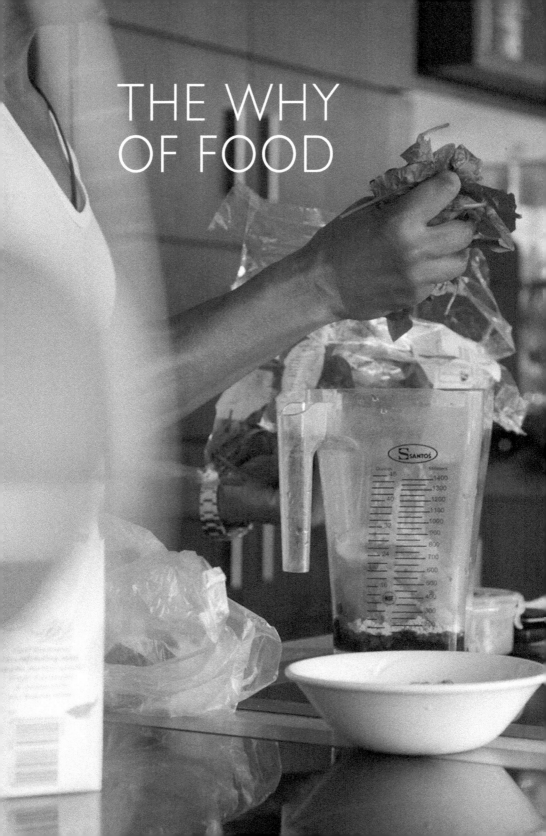

THE WHY
OF FOOD

# EATING FOR HEALTH

## OUR DIET... AND WHAT WE PUT IN OUR MOUTHS...

WE'RE NOT ALL the same shape – life would be very dull if we were – but body shaming and pressure on young girls through social media is increasingly rife; and the strain that being overweight puts on our bodies and general health is well documented – even if the best and worst things to eat seem to fluctuate with fashions from one month to the next.

There is an ever-increasing level of hype and hysteria around our diets….with the bottom line being much the same as for exercise. We all want to live longer and look better. Back through time, many years ago, our bodies evolved to avoid starvation rather than cope with the then unheard of perils of overeating. Hence hunger signals are stronger than those that tell us to stop eating.

## FOOD, GLORIOUS FOOD

Over the past 100 years there has been an enormous shift in the types of food available – pre-processed and packaged food make our lives easier, but also often contain more calories, more additives, are bigger portions, and just 'more'…

So now we have reached the point where, despite famine in parts of the world, and children starving, one in three people in the world are overweight.

- 11 million people in the UK are on a diet at any one time

- 80% of those losing weight will put it back on again

Cravings and old habits tend to die hard. So what is needed is to break a bad food relationship and create NEW habits. Losing weight starts with a relatively simple equation:

*You have to burn up more calories than you consume.*

Sounds oh so simple? There have been studies done as to whether some people's genes make them more likely to be overweight, some have big bones, the bacteria in your gut (that breaks down your food) may be different to that of your friend and work more or less efficiently, etc. etc… but at the end of the day what you actually put in your mouth has a big influence on what shape you are.

We are apparently quite bad at gauging how much we eat. Hence if big plates are fashionable, we don't realise that we have put a lot more onto them (come back nouvelle cuisine, all is forgiven?) Similarly we are not mindful enough about what we eat…watching TV whilst we chew, checking our inbox and Facebook page with fork poised….we don't actually pay attention to what we put into our mouths. And, of course, the social sadness of texting in preference to talking over dinner is well known. Even teenagers have begun to feel bad and (occasionally) put their phones in a pile and opt instead to talk to each other over coffee.

## FOCUS ON WHAT YOU WANT YOUR LIFE TO LOOK LIKE, NOT JUST YOUR BODY…

Culture tries to dictate to us what a socially acceptable weight is, or an ideal body shape actually looks like…but ideal forms have changed over the years. There are campaigns and complaints about 'body shaming' ads, but even whilst slamming the advertising hoardings with unbelievably thin models and lauding those who are proud to be bigger, our obsession with weight continues…

Of course it isn't 'just' for appearance sake – keeping our weight under control is advisable for health reasons: to prevent a range of diseases such as heart disease and diabetes, as well as putting less strain on our joints and muscles used in keeping us upright and carrying us around.

The advertising agencies are on a roll – wholefoods / natural ingredients / low sugar / low fat / no fat / detox / organic / artisan – emblazon the right emotive word across the packaging and bump up the price. Get healthy quick. We are told how to do it and there are any number of foods which claim to be the quick fix, drawing us in with promises of eternal youth. Be careful though – natural sounds good, wholefood must be healthy, detox and organic are pretty trendy…but what about sugar, salt, butter etc. They are 'natural' ingredients too, and too much of any single one can have a detrimental effect on your health.

An 'experiment' carried out on a BBC programme *The Truth about Healthy Eating* gave an interesting take on how packaging, wording and our own preconceptions can trip us up. A supposed new brand of bottled water, labelled refreshing, detailing the pH balance, number of electrolytes and its essential qualities for human health was launched to an exercise group with free samples in attractive bottles. The group tried it and answered a questionnaire. They decreed it 12% more refreshing than other bottled waters, 6% better for hydrating, estimated it at 20% healthier and accepted a price of 95p per bottle (roughly twice the supermarket equivalent). They all liked the flavour…which just goes to show that Glasgow tap water tastes nice (the new brand was simply bottled tap water).

A healthy diet doesn't have to mean relinquishing all pleasures; there is a healthy balance. We need certain things in our diets, how much of them we need depends on what we do in our daily lives. It is generally acknowledged that we eat too much processed food now, that we eat too much full stop, that too much sugar is bad for you. It is starting to be pointed out that the things scientists have replaced sugar and salt with are also bad for you, if not worse. At the same time, though, we are all individuals and our body may react differently to that of our neighbour.

Wayne starts the day with his 'Super-Ager' smoothie, packed with vegetables and fruit and nuts and healthy stuff. But he drinks that because he likes it, and doesn't believe in deprivation as a diet. He is also happy to eat the occasional pizzas, burgers, fish, and chips when out with his son. Or to drink beer while watching the football, red wine with a meal and on special occasions a rum and coke every now and again.

He abstains when possible from foods deemed really unhealthy, but the odd deviation is permitted. We all need treats to keep us motivated; though not too many or too often.

## EVERYTHING IN MODERATION

Surely it used to work? An occasional TV dinner, an occasional meal out at the fast food burger place, an occasional chocolate cake with the whipped cream on top. It can't be bad for you as long as you exercise enough to work it off afterwards, right?

Wrong! It's not only what you weigh! Or how you look on the outside; as Wayne discovered when he did a full reactions test with a nutritionist.

Katie is a Nutritional Therapist, running one-to-one sessions for adults and children at her own clinic as well as 'Wellness at Work'workshops and talks in-house she was also the Nutritionist at Champneys Health Spa Resort in Tring, where Wayne underwent tests to see if his body was as healthy on the inside, as it looked on the outside. He took the Lorician Health Analysis test – and discovered that while his muscle tone and skin kept him looking great on the outside, things weren't working quite so well on the inside!

Your body reacts in different ways to different foodstuffs, so a diet that works wonders for your best friend may not suit you or work the way you imagine. Food intolerance tests will show the reaction of your body to specific foods at a particular moment in time. Katie stresses, though, the importance of recognizing that intolerance does not equal allergy.

Actual allergies are for life, but food intolerances can arise as a result of negative factors or elements combining at a specific moment – imbalances which build up in your system and are exacerbated by other factors such as stress, excessive consumption or a reaction with other foods. By cutting out certain foods that the body has taken against, you give it a chance to readjust – to calm down. The lining of the stomach (i.e. the epithelial cells) is replaced by the body approximately every five days. Eliminating problem foods for a little longer than that – about four to six months according to Katie – and then slowly reintroducing them, can solve the problem. Sixty-five percent of digestion issues that people suffer from are ongoing problems rather than insoluble ones.

Gene mapping – DNA screening – goes one step further and dictates your ideal foods through your DNA. It is specific and personalised, looking at 47 genes in your body in 13 key areas and producing a blueprint that doesn't change. It will tell you which are harmful and can cause other illnesses, such as IBS (irritable bowel syndrome), or which ones simply upset the balance of our bodies and don't quite 'agree' with us.

Wayne has had an ongoing stomach issue and the results of his test did not make pleasant reading among other things he discovered that he is lactose intolerant and has a 'leaky gut'. His body therefore reacts against a lot of processed and added sugar foods, and based on his results, Katie advised him to avoid dairy, yeast, beef and lamb as much as possible.

Wayne set on a new path to introduce better eating habits, recipes that are made without additives or processed foods. Coming to terms with the imbalances and intolerances that the tests had shown up was not easy.

**He tried to avoid:**

- Processed foods

- Preservatives and additives

- Foods with added sugars

- Fast foods

- Foods with high levels of bad fats (all trans/some saturated)

- Refined grains and sugars

Wayne observed that 'When I was hungry I was often eating without thinking, but my condition meant that I had to be mindful of what I was putting into my body. It's not easy because I do have naughty days – but boy, do I pay the price! My gut almost immediately knows when I have eaten badly. But life without the occasional burger and chips with either a beer or rum and Coke is very difficult.'

## KNOW THE CHANGE YOU WANT TO SEE

Inevitably some of the irritating items on Wayne's list do make their way into his diet sometimes, but as he puts it, 'Once you know the effect a particular food has on you, you alone have to weigh up the negative effects on your stomach, or your body as a whole, against your enjoyment of it; and decide on a balance.'

Research has shown that people who are generally 'into' healthier eating are more concerned about being healthy as a way of preventing disease, rather than looking to overcome a specific one. Often though, people eliminate everyday foods from their diet to be generally healthier and find that a long-term problem also goes away. This has happened with hay fever, and others who've suffered with arthritis have had similar results. The proven added benefits of healthy eating include increased immunity and energy levels, a decrease in allergies and improved blood sugar and overall mood, and an increased feeling of general wellbeing.

In the same way as we learn a new exercise routine and make it part of our daily lives, so certain foods that we know do us good and also make us feel good (physically, or mentally, or both…'look at me, eating healthily!') can become accepted as a natural part of the new you. People are often lulled into a false sense of security when their figure is more or less ok.

Ultimately you have to look both inside and out, treating the whole body in order to see the whole picture and change for the better.

*'You can't exercise your way out of a bad diet.'*

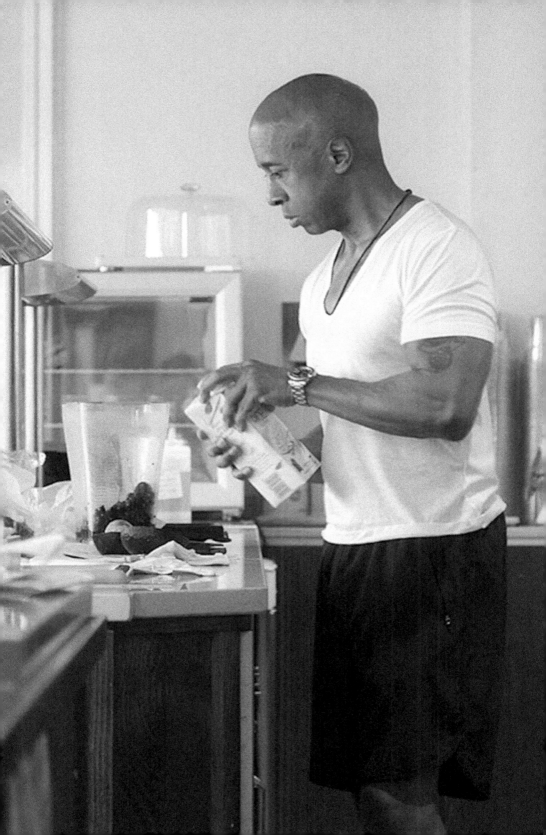

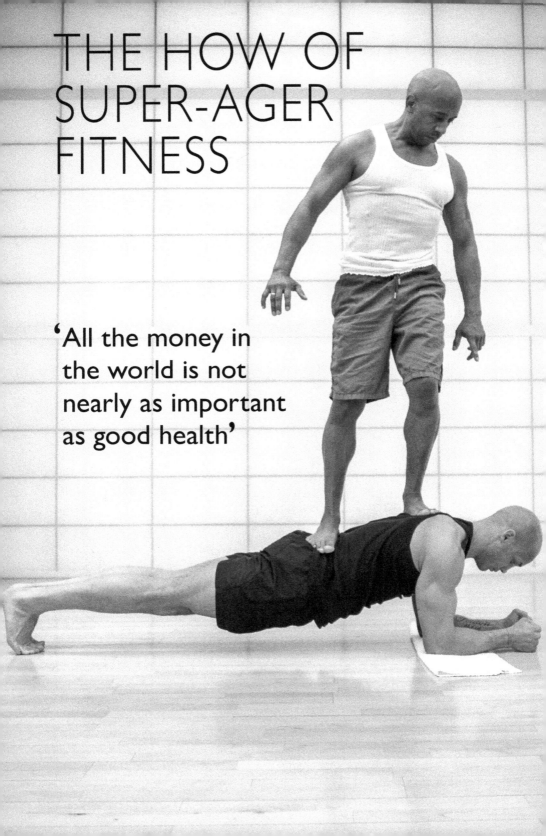

# THE HOW OF SUPER-AGER FITNESS

'All the money in the world is not nearly as important as good health'

# BECOMING A SUPER-AGER

- **Embrace mental challenges:** for the sense of achievement and self-fulfilment.

- **Exercise regularly:** develop self-discipline and, in turn, enhance many other aspects of your life.

- **Practise mindfulness:** reinforce your ability to be intensely aware – of yourself and your surroundings.

SUPER-AGER FITNESS is not just a workout for the body, it also influences your mind and emotions. It is based on a 35-year empirical study that conceptualises the process of intentional behavioural change (if you don't know where you are going, how will you know when you get there?). It works alongside two innovative exercise programmes: JumpGa and Kun-Aqua; aimed at intelligent people, 35 and above who want to preserve their youth right down to their DNA.

In your 20s you took your body for granted. In your 30s you started to know your body better, and what it was capable of. In your 40s gravity, hormones, slowing metabolism, decreased lean muscle mass and body fat increases occurred. Now it's about rewiring your body. This can lead to successful change because your body can be convinced to improve itself through self-belief; using the Transtheoretical Model of Behavioural Change (TTM) as a guide to developing a more disciplined approach.

## THE THEORY – THE STAGES OF CHANGE

Scientists have done numerous behavioural studies and come up with a logical set of stages that each person passes through on their way to making positive changes to their behaviour – whether it be losing weight, increasing exercise or stopping smoking. These have been concluded after 35 years of scientific research and empirical studies and amalgamated into one theoretical model covering a variety of scenarios and social factors. It is called the Transtheoretical Model of Behavioural Change (TTM).

The Stages of Change lie at the heart of the TTM. Studies of change have found that people move through a series of stages when modifying behaviour. The amount of time it takes to pass from one stage to another varies, of course, depending on the change in question and the individual undertaking it – but the factors or things to be completed in order to pass from one stage to another remain fixed. Certain principles and processes of change work best at each stage to reduce resistance, facilitate progress, and prevent relapse. These include decisional balance, self-efficacy, and processes of change. Only a minority (usually less than 20%) of a population at risk is prepared to take action at any given time. Thus, action-oriented guidance (the traditional tool of change) mis-serves individuals in the early stages. Guidance based on the TTM results in increased participation in the change process because it appeals to the whole population rather than the minority ready to take action.

One critical acknowledgment behind TTM is that change is occurring over a period of time. Traditionally, behaviour change was often seen as an event, such as quitting smoking, drinking, or overeating. TTM recognises change as a process that unfolds over time, involving progress through a series of stages. While progression through the Stages of Change can occur in a linear fashion; one after the other, individuals often retrace their steps, falling back to earlier stages from later ones.

So change is not a one-off event: it is a process, a series of small movements and slight adjustments. Those small changes are what can ultimately get you from where you are now to where you want to be. This scientific study fixed the stages we go through as we give up a bad habit or take on board a new one.

### Precontemplation (Not Ready)

People in the Precontemplation stage don't recognise a need for change and are often unaware (either uninformed or under informed) that their behaviour or situation is problematic or has negative consequences. They do not intend to take action in the foreseeable future, usually measured as the next six months.

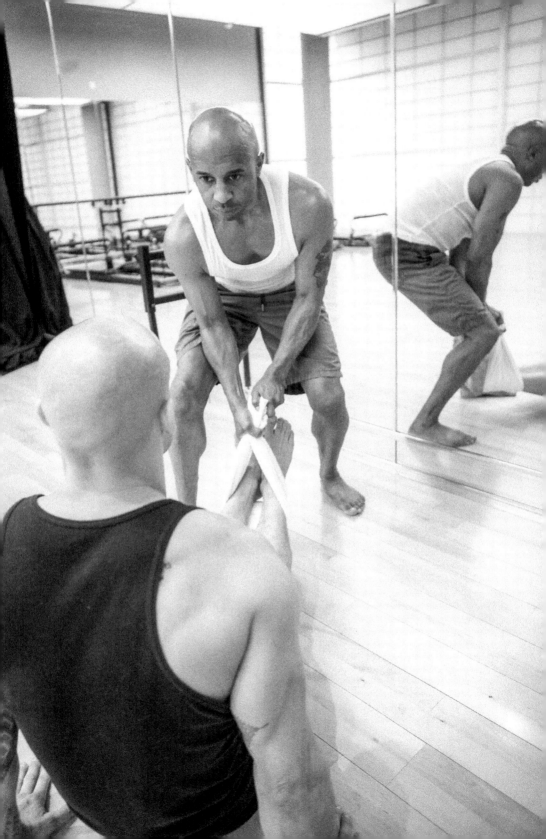

People at this stage may also be demoralised by previous attempts that failed and consider themselves unable to change.

### Contemplation (Getting Ready)

Contemplation is the stage in which people are aware of the need to alter, but not committed to taking action. They do intend to change, in the next six months, and are aware of both the pros and cons of the action. If they consider them more or less equal, people can stay at this stage for a long period of time.

### Preparation (Ready)

This is the point where 'I should' changes to 'I will'. Preparation is the stage in which people intend to take action in the immediate future, usually measured as the next month. Typically, they already have a plan of action, such as joining a health education class, consulting a counsellor, talking to their physician, buying a self-help book, or relying on a self-change approach.

### Action (Starting off)

Action is the stage in which people have changed their behaviour or modified their lifestyles – attending a workshop, joining a gym, starting an exercise programme, and made specific overt modifications in their lifestyles within the past six months. Because action is a visual state rather than a thought or plan, the overall process of behaviour change has often been equated with action, but in the TTM, Action is only one of six stages!

### Maintenance (Keeping it up)

People in this stage have made specific modifications in their lifestyles and are working to prevent relapse. While in this stage (defined as when people have kept up their new habits for more than six months), people grow increasingly more confident that they can sustain the changes they have made and will work hard to avoid relapse.

### Termination (Achievement)

At this stage, the new habits have been incorporated into a lifestyle and the individual will continue with their behaviour (in this case exercise and wellbeing) regardless of what life throws at them. Whether depressed, anxious, bored, lonely, angry, or stressed, individuals in this stage are sure they will not return to unhealthy habits as a way of coping. It is as if their new behaviour has become an automatic habit. In reality, this stage – 100% self-efficacy, where nothing can shake your new habits - is seldom reached and people tend to stay in 'maintenance'.

### Tipping the Scales

The whole decision-making process that goes into the change in behaviour, the taking up of a new habit, was conceptualized by Janis and Mann (1977) as a decisional 'balance sheet' of comparative potential gains and losses that influence moves from one stage to another. Two components of this decisional balance, the pros and the cons, have become critical in the Transtheoretical Model. As individuals progress through the Stages of Change, the gains or advantages to be gained from change must become greater than the losses, so that there is an incentive to keep moving on and sustain the new behaviour (i.e. the exercise, or the diet, or the non-smoking). As the scales tip, so a habit is formed…

**Motivation gets you started, habit keeps you going…**

The Transtheoretical Model of Behavioural Change serves as an important guide in the process of behavioural change, of altering your lifestyle and is the rationale behind the Super-Ager programme. Wayne didn't devise the theory, but he lived it, and his training programme mirrors the steps within it.

Each stage is a benchmark to measure yourself against, or for Wayne to measure his clients. It helps him in the search for a goal, acting as a tool to outline and develop a strategy specific to that person's needs. In the same way, it can help you individually to assess where you are, why you are there, and where you are going next.

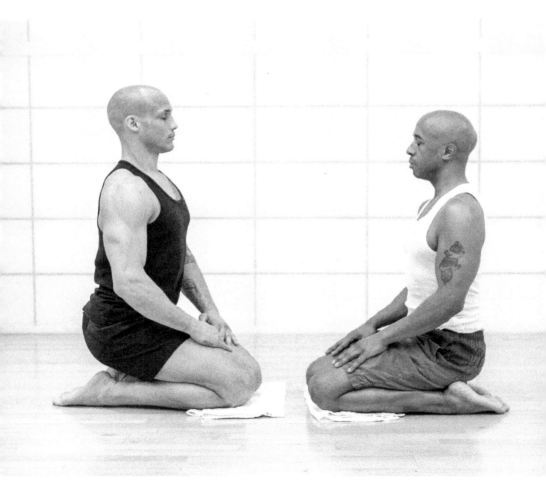

# THE PRACTICE – AGELESS TRANSFORMATION

Sounds ideal? It is. Sounds too good to be true? It isn't! It is achievable – if you want it enough. Why do we exercise? Why do we so desperately want to change the way we look?

We long to stay trim, get thin, keep fit, feel better, lose weight and look simply stunning – all in order to improve ourselves, or some aspect of ourselves, in our eyes, or the eyes of other people around us.

We want to lose weight, look good, live more healthily and for longer. Hence the gym memberships, the New Year resolutions, the designer trainers. But if it doesn't last then the frustration can set you back, and many people eventually give up all together rather than face the seesaw of weight, energy, and emotion…

So? Find an exercise routine that works for you; that is geared around your lifestyle and shows results. Find one that actually makes you feel and look better. 'Ah, but better than what?' The world is so preoccupied with perfection, but it comes in different forms. Fashion companies throw photos of perfect models at us – but they are photo-shopped images, not real people and certainly not a vision to aim for. In fact, social media is a dangerous source of role models – research found that people (particularly teenagers) check their social media accounts upwards of 120 minutes per day (sounds like a lot, but add your minutes up and see) and they are twice as likely to develop eating disorders and body image concerns.

As we get older, we like to think we are less at the mercy of others, less prone to needing approval in the way we look or lead our lives. The over-40s are (according to a 25-year University of Alberta study) no longer people-pleasers and are more willing and able to take ownership of their lives. Add to that the fact that the perfect body image has radically altered over the years and there really is not a single specific shape that we should all be working towards.

We can all feel good about ourselves though; take control of our bodies and minds and maximise their potential. We can sculpt our own shapes a little and be the best that we possibly can. A role model can really help too – someone who models the habits you want to mirror. You may not want the same muscles as them but if their determination and focus helps you with yours, it'll probably be a beautiful friendship.

A 'want-to goal' is proven to achieve greater success. So, a goal for everyone, but not the same goal… You have to decide what it is you want to achieve: how much weight you want to lose, how much muscle you want to build, how much better you want to feel. Fix your own personal 'want' for exercise and make it a really strong desire. You need to have a powerful motivating force to carry you along, but you also need something recognisable when you get there. Wayne's goal is to be able to fit the same size and style of T-shirt that he has worn for years, saying: 'My body metric is a comfortable -fitting white T-shirt, it is my guide to not let genetics and ageing take control'.

Wayne's training involves a series of small psychological and physical changes rather than one giant leap. It is the magic combination of an exercise regime that is 'do-able' at all levels with one that actually works – if you keep at it! It has an 80% higher success rate than joining a gym in terms of 'start, stick at it and get a result' and a unique 3-step strategy to start you off towards improved body image, self-esteem, and self-confidence.

# WAYNE'S 3-STEP STRATEGY

## STEP 1. THE GOAL

Setting the right goals can lead to successful change. Fitness is a variable concept and cannot be reached without effort – so it is important to set SMART goals, i.e. Specific, Measurable, Achievable, Realistic, Time-frame goals to work towards. Once you have set that long-term goal in your mind and accepted that it requires mental and physical change, it will always be there. Break down the negativity – move your body and change your mind. All the steps are there to change the way you feel, look, think and communicate. Remember to make the goal realistic: something you really want; enough to fight your shortcomings, your down days, and anyone else's obstacles; something that you want to keep doing. Visualising how you want to look and feel in the future will have to become your everyday thinking, as if it's already happened. As with any process, repeating the thoughts and actions over and over again will stop the mind debating whether it can be done; you will simply accept that it will be done.

Take a piece of paper and spend a little time answering the following questions:

- What's your goal?

- Where are you now?

- How will you feel when you have it?

- How will you know when you have it?

- When do you want it?

- What do you need to achieve your goal?

- For what purpose do you want this?

- What will you gain or lose if you have it?

- What will happen if you get it?

- What will happen if you don't get it?

## STEP 2. THE METHOD

Pick the best programme. What Wayne offers is the perfect metaphor for change because learning a new exercise routine involves a mental process – the same process we use for everything we do in daily life. Once you have learned each exercise there is a mental concept of its outcome – a visual memory of the movement, and the breath (inhale or exhale) that comes with it, and an internal dialogue, telling yourself what comes next. Once you experience and understand the mental process of learning a new routine it can easily be broken down and applied to other aspects of life where you need a little extra self-confidence or success.

## STEP 3. REINFORCEMENT

The mindfulness, or state of relaxation, associated with assimilating new lessons and reinforcing your belief in yourself is a crucial factor in successful exercise, no matter which exercise programme you choose to follow. Mindfulness is quite simply the ability to be intensely aware of yourself and your surroundings, to the extent of being able to detach yourself from current locations or situations. Every minute of every day, your body is reacting physically to what is happening mentally; literally changing and responding to the thoughts that are going through your mind. A thought is actually an electro-chemical event that is taking place in your nerve cells and then producing a whole cascade of physiological changes.

Your life doesn't change the genes that you were born with, but things that happen to you in your life do alter your genetic activity – as in all the chemicals in your body that regulate your cell. So in a sense, you are 'speaking' to your genes with every thought that you have. The good news is that the cells in your body are replaced roughly every two months, so you can re-programme cells to be more optimistic by adopting positive thinking practices. Every thought of yours is a thing that influences other things and, by channelling them, you really can change yourself and your life.

Be firm but realistic. When you resolve to start training, start small, and commit to just 21 days of training. You need a control mechanism. Put a rubber band or bracelet onto your wrist. If you miss a day, simply move the band or bracelet onto your other wrist and start counting again from the beginning!

Wayne's previous book was called '20-21' – and advocated 20 minutes of exercise per day for 21 days. Why 21 days? Because after that time the results should be visible in terms of shape, strength, and flexibility, and the positive habit hopefully on its way to being formed; so that exercise becomes an instinct, a part of the daily routine rather than something to drag yourself along to.

Try it – choose your goal and then invest 21 days of your life in starting off along the path towards it. Rewire your own beliefs and thoughts about yourself.

## THE TRAINING

Often people who rush into a new exercise programme after a long lay-off can become more susceptible to sprains, pulled muscles, fractures, shin splints and other injuries; overdoing it in a sudden burst of enthusiasm.

**Super-Ager** Fitness reduces stress, the risk of injury and decreases muscle tension and weakness. It helps people meet their mental, weight and fitness goals, building focus, strength, endurance, and flexibility. At the same time it pays attention to awareness, form, and functional movement in order to address mind and body imbalances with primary, basic movement patterns that also combat age-related changes. It avoids the 'one size fits all' theory. Exercises are adapted to your fitness levels and targets, to your starting point and where you want to get – to determine the combination and intensity of the exercises.

Fads and fashions come and go, but there are exercise elements that have stood the test of time. Martial Arts practices date back thousands of years – emphasising intense control of mind and body in their sequences of movements. Wayne's programme draws on those movements, particularly in its Kun-Aqua and JumpGa programmes; combining the Eastern philosophy of meditative movement with the Western expertise in dynamic, aerobic exercise.

The ultimate aim of Super-Ager Fitness is to effectively relax the mind and recruit the deep stabilising muscles to control the position of the spine during dynamic movements. The emphasis is on doing only a few simple movements to bring awareness into what you do, as this is far more important than rushing through a series of exercises.

Performing a pre work-out body scan is a mental technique used to increase awareness of physical sensations and to help you get in touch with your body. By paying attention to physical sensations, you can more easily cease the constant barrage of thoughts that can interfere with attempts to meditate. The body scan is best performed before your workout or during your warm-up, although certain parts of this technique can be practised any time you feel your mind start to wander. Begin by standing still, allowing your awareness to settle into your body. Take a few deep breaths. Mentally scan your body to see if you have any places of tightness or pain, breathing into these areas to release the tension. A formal body scan involves lying on the ground and rotating your consciousness throughout various parts of your body, focusing on one particular muscle group at a time. You may wish to perform the formal body scan after your exercise programme to bring closure to your meditation practice.

## KUN-AQUA

Kun-Aqua Water exercise is for the Wise Man. Up to 65% of the adult body is made of water and every living cell in the body needs it to keep functioning. The non-swimming water exercises improve mobility and strength, increase circulation, rehabilitate healing muscles, control body weight and reduce wear on joints.

**The practice of Kun-Aqua entails three key components:**

**Movement** – fluid movements improve the body's alignment. Posture, strength, flexibility, co-ordination, balance, and stamina are all increased. Many of these benefits of Kun-Aqua are

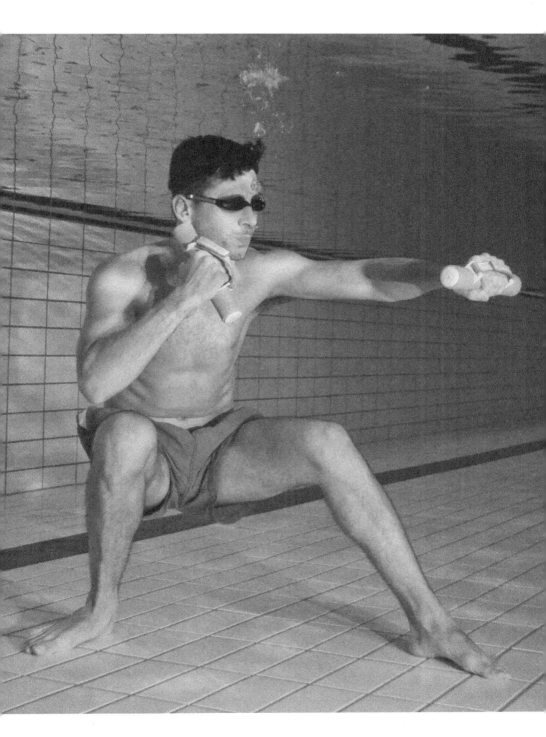

consistent with other forms of low impact exercise, but Kun-Aqua offers the added benefit of focus on improved posture, balance, and alignment.

**Breathing** – rhythmical, focused breathing emphasises control, opens the airways, and encourages strong oxygenated blood circulation to the muscles and brain.

**Meditation/a state of mind** – practitioners have said that they experience a meditative state of mind during Kun-Aqua training; that the concentration on movements and breathing helps to dissipate stress and anxiety caused by external factors.

If you have ever tried to quickly to get out of a pool, then you will understand the difficulty of moving fast in water. The non-swimming water exercises can also seriously shake up your workout routine and break free of the monotony of the gym by getting into the water.

The Mayo Clinic confirms that training in water is the ultimate resistance exercise; unique, because it's low impact (your body is supported by the water), but simultaneously intense because of the water resistance. Every action involves more effort due to the natural instability of the water and increased resistance since you are pushing against the density of water, rather than against air. It is deemed the best exercise environment for all abilities and levels of fitness.

*Motion is the thing that turns on muscles, not the mind.*

Kun-Aqua comprises two new exercise programmes: one drawing on ancient healing techniques of mindfulness-based movement in the water; and the other on the more modern idea of power training in water. One is a slow and deliberate walking practice that requires the student to be tranquil and calm during focused movements. The other is an athletic, high-calorie burning, strength and power discipline.

**The overall physical benefits of Kun-Aqua are:**

- Physically, it is a total body workout requiring incredible activation and stabilisation of all your muscles. You can burn 30 percent more calories than you would by practising the same workout on land.

- Lack of flexibility is more easily resolved in water-based exercise because it is much easier to move your joints through their full range of motion and reach full extension in water without stressing them.

- Water provides more resistance than air and is the perfect place to get fit. You work your heart, tone your muscles and build your strength faster and more effectively than on dry land. All whilst giving your joints a rest, and minimising any risk of injury.

- Over 60 percent of your body weight is water. Gravity and body weight impacts on the way the body moves.

- Water has the added benefit of hydrating, oxygenating and revitalizing the body's musculo-skeletal system. The effect of gravitational pull is removed, and weightlessness qualities are achieved. The range of movement increases; and repetition, stretching, and balancing is more sustainable.

- The heart pumps more rigorously when the body is submerged. Hydrostatic pressure – or the pressure in water at rest due to the weight of the water above that point – provides benefits by decreasing swelling, reducing blood pressure and improving joint position. This, in turn, improves your proprioception, or body awareness.

- If you work out whilst in water up to neck level, your body weight is effectively reduced by as much as 90 percent. A 9st 4lb woman working out neck deep in water would weigh less than a stone, putting much less strain on her body.

- Kun-Aqua burns about 30 percent more calories than the equivalent exercise on land. Since water offers 12–18 times more resistance than air, muscles are given a workout from every angle — resulting in greater muscle definition and all-around strength.

- Training in water disperses body heat about four times faster than air at the same temperature, naturally helping to maintain the core body temperature within an acceptable range, and preventing the overheating common with vigorous, land-based exercise.

'Calories burned: Water-walking or jogging burns 563 calories per hour if you weigh 155 pounds, and 654 calories an hour if you weigh 180 pounds. Water-running burns 11.5 calories per minute in comparison with running on land, which burns about 8 calories per minute', according to The Sunday Times (22 November 2010).

## KUN-AQUA – THE MENTAL

Being in the present moment is an act of mindfulness – of simply paying attention to what is. You can become the non-judgmental observer of whatever feelings and thoughts may arise without the need to take action. Kun-Aqua walking meditation promotes the ability to witness the movement without attachment to the sensations in your body, and any feelings or thoughts you may have.

Breath awareness is a critical component of meditation. Paying special attention to the way you breathe, will help you take the focus off your thoughts and worries. Simply tune into your breathing patterns, and observe the flow of breath without judgment or criticism. Your inhalation should come from your abdominal area, for a complete slow breath.

Focus on the control of your breath – it is at that moment you will become aware of the magic starting to happen. The mind will become quieter and a calm awareness arises. Doing the movements alone, without actively involving the breath, is like singing a song without rhythm.

As a result of the calm awareness, emotional stress and random thoughts are less likely to occur. Your energy will begin to flow more freely; pushing through any emotional and physical blockages and thus freeing the body and mind, which results in the post-workout 'feel good' effect.

Breath has everything to do with your structural alignment and the patterns in which you perceive and move your body. Breath awareness can eliminate joint compression and other imbalances from your posture and attitude. Awareness of breath in the water practice is the same foundation for flowing seamlessly in movement through a yoga practice.

## KUN-AQUA – THE PHYSICAL

Having had several knee and hip surgeries along with low back pain issues Wayne's exercise choices were limited. He discovered that walking backwards in water required less range of motion, less strain on the knee joints, improved his pelvic alignment that helped open up the facet joints in his spine and reduce compression that was causing his low back pain. The water's buoyancy also allowed for more pain-free movement. Wayne believes that his programme can be of great benefit to the medical profession and employers at a time when a series of studies published in *The Lancet* names lower back pain as the leading cause of disability in the world.

## KUN-AQUA – KYPHOSIS PREVENTION

Curvature of the spine, is most common in women between the ages of 50 and 70 due to having a higher risk for osteoporosis. If unchecked, there is a decline in physical functioning with detrimental effects on the ability to perform everyday activities of daily living, and quality of life. Kun-Aqua exercises can improve postural alignment and strengthen back muscles to counteract the forward pull on the spine, and delay the progress of kyphosis.

## KUN-AQUA – EXERCISE EFFICIENCY

Water provides natural resistance in all directions, strengthening the abdominal muscles that stabilise the body, to maintain balance as it reacts to the turbulence and buoyancy of the water surrounding you. Resistance determines your intensity. By increasing your speed, you increase the intensity of the workout. The higher the water level, the more challenging the workout.

## KUN-AQUA – EYES SHUT

Performing KUN-AQUA movements with your eyes closed can help enhance how it feels and allow you to better tap into your mind–muscle connection (MMC). This enables you to better remember body position, joint angles, the degree of muscular tension, and movement patterns.

The visual cortex doesn't close down when you close your eyes because it is still active, imagining visual images. When you think of a yoga pose with your eyes closed your visual cortex is recruited in order for you to visualise what the pose looks like, possibly improving focus, mental acuity and the ability to perform an action independently of visual information.

## KUN-AQUA – BACKWARD WALKING

Moving backward in water works your muscles and joints in different ways from forward walking. It elicits the greatest muscle activation of the entire three layers of the intrinsic back muscles, which are located beneath two more superficial back muscle groups that together make up the extrinsic back muscles. These muscles extend your spine and bend it over to the same side on which the contracting muscle is located. People with on-going or recurrent episodes of lower back pain should consider the benefits of walking in water.

## HOW-TO

Kun-Aqua walking backward routine will help you learn what it feels like to be mindful while doing an activity you already know. To begin, stand in an upright position with shoulders back, chest lifted and arms bent slightly at your sides. Practise the body scan and pay attention to your breathing. Focus on your surroundings and the sensations in and around your body. Slowly stride backward, placing the ball of your foot on the bottom of the pool, followed by your whole foot. Avoid straining your back by keeping your core (stomach and back muscles) engaged as you walk. Feel the way your body and arms movement work against the water resistance as you propel yourself backward. Love the experience of movement, release the tension in your shoulders and neck. Avoid the tendency to lean back into the water; instead,  maintain a straight back and draw your abdominal muscles inwards to keep yourself upright.

## KUN-AQUA – SUMMARY

Kun-Aqua is a total body workout requiring incredible mental activation and stabilisation of all your muscles to keep you upright and breathing regularly and to propel you through the water. It is also a soothing, contemplative practice where close attention is paid to the action of movement. This is about being mindful of your muscle recruitment and the placement of the feet, balance, and motion.  Kun-Aqua is a method by which to rehabilitate, or re-educate, the human body; as you become mindful of the movement of each step. Simply moving back and forth between the calm and turbulence of water will increase your ability to focus and to keep yourself fully present in the moment. Wayne has learned from experience: trying out and perfecting his programmes whilst training himself and clients, who include top sportsmen and captains of industry.

## REBOUNDING

Remember the fun of jumping on the bed? Rebounding – 'trampolining' for the beginners amongst us – is a low impact, full body, weight-bearing exercise that ensures optimal health and fitness. The rebounders

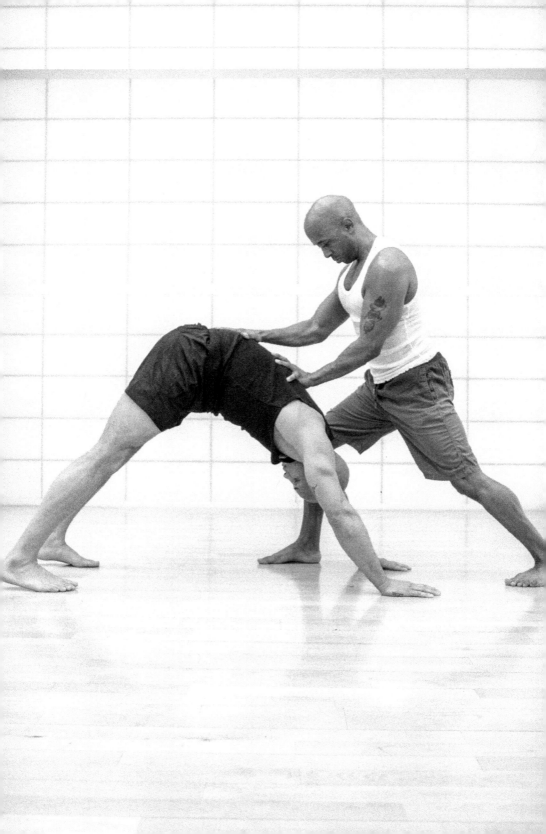

removes up to 85% of the impact that your joints would otherwise experience if you did the same sets of exercises (star jumps, squats, running on the spot) on solid ground. And since, logically, you work harder on a springy surface than a solid one, such as a treadmill, you burn up 100 more calories for every 10 minutes you spend bouncing up and down. NASA scientists have described it as 'the most efficient and effective exercise known to man' – and they know a thing or two about the effects of weightlessness!

As you are weightless for a few seconds at the top of each bounce, the gravitational pull that comes into force as you come down again multiplies the resistance, puts all the cells and muscles under a consistent rhythmic pressure and hence strengthens and tones the entire body.

All this adds up to building muscle without putting too much strain on the body; strengthening your core and improving your posture and balance – if you don't focus and stay concentrated you can rebound off in the wrong direction (and yes, that's the voice of experience talking). It's definitely 'mindful' training, not mindless; as well as being fantastic fun!

## REBOUNDING AND BONE STRENGTH

Our skeleton is the scaffolding that supports us against the forces of gravity and resists the pull of the muscles to allow movement. Bone is a living tissue that has its own blood vessels and changes over the course of a lifetime. This process is called remodelling, where new bone cells replace older or damaged bone cells. Scientists estimate that through this process, the skeleton completely remodels itself every ten years. By the age of 30, however, people generally achieve maximum bone density and strength (peak bone mass). Thereafter, our bone density gradually begins to decline as we age. It's not all doom and gloom though; because a healthy diet and exercise, particularly exercise like rebounding (weight-bearing and resistance movements rolled into one), are a natural way to build bones. Rebounding can slow the bone reduction that usually occurs as we age and protect bone health in older adults, including those with low bone density (osteoporosis); which may in turn help to reduce the risk of our bones breaking.

## REBOUNDING AND MUSCLE STRENGTH

Muscle burns calories even when you are resting, so it is important to maintain muscle mass. From the age of 35, you begin to lose muscle mass and fat levels increase, so you are burning fewer calories and the ageing process is accelerating. The decline is relatively slow and steady at first but, it accelerates as you age.

Because the process of muscle loss is so gradual, you are not fully aware that your body is changing. An increase in fat typically hides the muscle loss; making you less likely to notice what's happening. When people do realise that their body has changed from a lean, slim torso to a less defined 'butter bean' shape, albeit one that can still fit into the same jeans; their muscle tone is no longer what it once was. This process will continue and over the course of time, you will add as much as 3lb of fat every year unless you change your diet or do more exercise. The more overweight and unhealthy you become, the more discouraging the thought of doing exercise will be; forming a vicious circle of defeat and poor health.

## REBOUNDING AND INTERNAL SYSTEMS

You need regular exercise and movement to ensure that your lymph system is effectively carrying nutrients to the cells, and waste products away from them. Without adequate movement, the cells are undernourished and left with waste products and this state contributes to arthritis, cancer and other degenerative diseases, as well as ageing.

When you bounce you are stimulating all of your internal organs, moving the cerebral-spinal fluid, and benefiting your intestines. You are also subjecting the body to gravitational pulls ranging from zero at the top of each bounce to two to three times the force of gravity at the bottom, depending on how high you are rebounding. This means

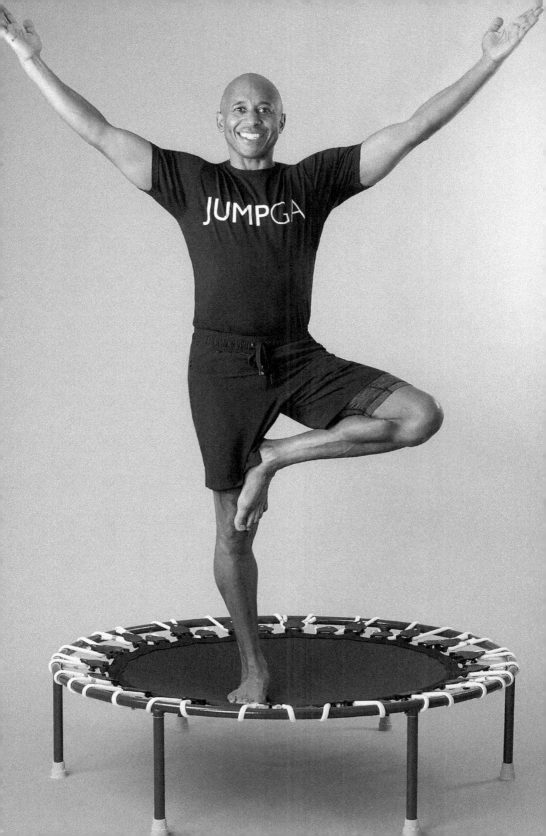

oxygen is flooding your cells, and your joints are under no strain, which makes it ideal for the elderly, overweight or unfit.

## YOGA ASANA

Yoga differs from more traditional gym-based or aerobic exercise, where the idea seems to be to go at it as hard as you can for as long as you can! It blends moves that improve circulation, balance, flexibility, and strength with meditative techniques that require controlled breathing. Yoga involves binding each breath to a movement; challenging your co-ordination and concentration. A short sequence of poses forms an exercise routine that will stretch and strengthen muscles and calm a wandering mind. You focus on your breath and clear your head of everyday worries and preoccupations – hence relieving stress, which in turn improves your overall mood. There has been a surge of women, particularly more mature ones, but of all shapes and sizes, signing up for yoga classes. But one has to be careful. One of my clients, Helen, had this to say about her experience.

*Stretching out to the goal of enlightenment...*

"I signed up for yoga classes – in different studios in different countries at different moments in my life; always twisting as best I could and thinking that the odd twinge the next day meant I wasn't stretching quite the right way or quite enough. Eventually, Wayne pointed out to me, gently but unequivocally, that different exercises fit different purposes and different people, and we are not all equally flexible. My aches and lower back pain didn't mean that I was doing the pose wrong, or should be pushing towards greater flexibility…it meant that maybe I shouldn't be pushing that way at all. Forward Asana, for instance, is perhaps not a pose that reflects a natural, physical movement in our daily lives. The message is 'don't force it'. Recognise and accept that not all bodies are made the same and if it hurts, don't do it – pain is not always gain!"

Some bodies are just inherently less 'flexible' than others. There are many studies, and the evidence from them suggests that a weekly diet of yoga and meditation may strengthen your thinking skills and help to ward off age-related mental decline. Inevitably our brains do weaken somewhat with age, but we may be able to slow the decline by altering how we live and, in particular, whether and how we move our bodies. A study by the *European Journal of Preventative Cardiology* back in 2014 found yoga just as effective as other more strenuous cardiovascular exercises at reducing the risk of heart disease. And of course, there are the long-accepted benefits of increased strength, improved muscle tone and greater flexibility; not to mention the bonus of being low impact, and hence kind to your bones and joints.

We are told in lots of yoga books that the Sanskrit word 'yoga' means 'union'. This is only half the truth. Its closest literal equivalent in the English language is 'yoke'. So yoga is really the art of yoking the 'lower' (or ego) personality to the 'higher' truth; of disciplining the combination of body and mind so that it becomes fitted to reality. Thus yoga signifies both the state of harmony and the means to realise it.

Adding Yoga Asana into the exercise mix shifts the focus to flexibility and breathing; to boost physical and mental wellbeing. It becomes a whole body workout that simultaneously strengthens your heart and lungs, boosts your immune system, and tones and flexes the muscles.

## JUMPGA

The fitness yoga fusion, to create an entirely new exercise plan.

Louise Day, the Director of Wellness at the UK's Number 1 spa, Champneys, said: *'I see more fitness choices available than ever before. HIIT or resistance workouts? Calisthenics or virtual boxing? Wellness or mindfulness? Group fitness classes have evolved markedly in recent years, and this is reflected in the wide range of group classes we offer. My job is to choose a training programme that has a future and will impact on people's physical and mental fitness. I see JumpGa as the complete training programme that will take exercise to a new level: because it's a total body programme that can be adapted to all ages and levels of fitness'.*

Wayne's JUMPGA programme is an industry first and a totally new way to look at a fitness class. It gives time-pushed exercisers the chance to leave early, arrive late, or do the whole class, once they have paid for their spot.

People are more likely to stick with an exercise programme when they don't have to spend hours in the gym. The JUMPGA Express class is based on the concept that even if someone is too busy to build in a regular 1-hour training session they can go for the JUMPGA express session instead.

It is a classic 10-minute HIIT workout that merges circuit training, yoga and functional training into one. It builds into a 45-minute workout that is perfect for burning fat and building muscle. The fixed sequence programme will be repeated three/four times (just like doing sets in weight training) during the 45-minute class. This enables people who can't to do a full-length class to do one, two or all of the sets, as they are broken down into 10-minute chunks.

JumpGa has enabled Wayne to rebuild his body to peak condition; achieving the body composition of an athlete. He says that doing this workout once or twice a week will help you burn MORE calories when you're doing the cardio section, because your muscles require more energy. The resulting increase in your metabolic rate after a JumpGa session can last for up to 24 hours. During this period after exercise, your body continues the accelerated breakdown of sugars and fats, the processing of oxygen, and the building of muscle – no matter what else you do. Every challenge forces us to search for a new centre of gravity. Don't fight it, just find a different way to stand.

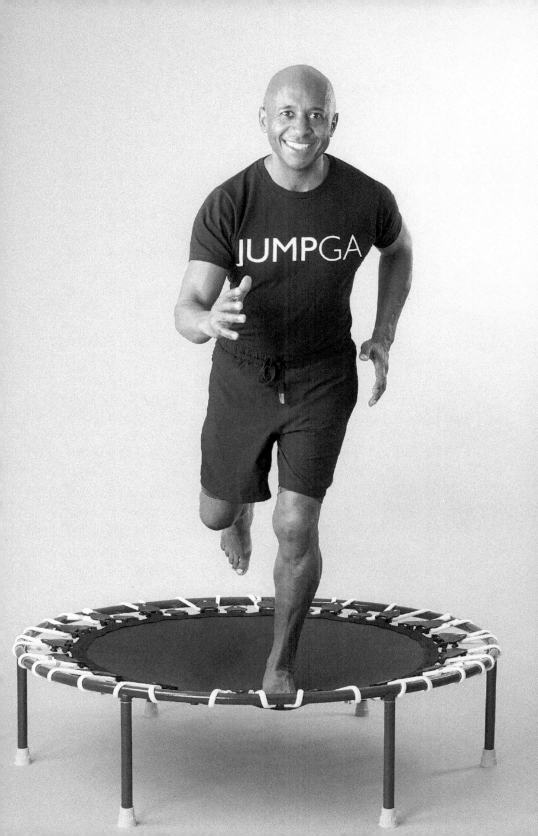

# JUMPGA – BACK-FRIENDLY PRACTICE

With an estimated one in ten people worldwide suffering from low back pain there has never been a better time to rethink the way that we exercise. The more you are able to twist into the postures (in some cases to contort), the better you assume yourself to be…but if it's not a pose echoing a necessary, natural movement of our bodies then are we better in ourselves for performing it? Stuart McGill, leading back pain researcher, maintains that we are not –that science has come up with no concrete benefit to increasing spine flexibility. Furthermore, some people are simply more flexible than others, depending on the genes you were born with, i.e. 'life isn't always fair' and some of us have to accept that we are 'flexion intolerant'!

JumpGa is a back-friendly practice. The Asana sequences bind your breath with every movement to develop a connection to your core and vertical alignment. They are a series of postures that mirror functional body movements that we make in the course of our everyday actions; promoting mobility, flexibility, strength and muscle suppleness.

How we feel manifests from the result of our hard work – you can feel when your exercise programme starts to reap rewards: the increase to your confidence that will result from moving towards your goal; the increase to your sense of health and wellbeing, perhaps a change to your figure that boosts your self-esteem. All of these positive changes will fire you with enthusiasm, and the resolve to keep going; to fulfil your goal and make a lasting change in yourself, your health and the way you feel.

The exercises aren't alternatives, or all compulsory! They can combine in different ways depending on age, your level of fitness, and of course what you ultimately want to achieve. They are interchangeable, so there is no monotony! All of them are aerobic and work on strength, flexibility, suppleness, and balance – but are simultaneously low impact, involve the element of mindfulness that strengthens the mind as well as the body and makes your exercise programme work and carry on working as a lifestyle change.

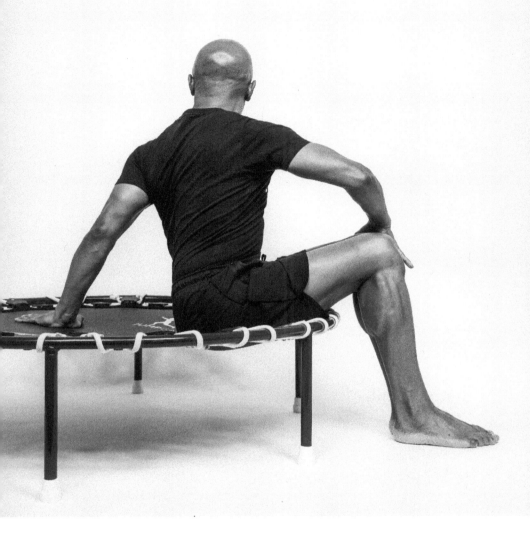

Learning and performing repetitions of exercises builds a pattern, which in turn forms a habit; so that exercising becomes an integral part of your daily life. The great news for calorie counters is that rebounding puts the numbers firmly on your side. If you weigh 75 kilos and go for a 30-minute jog, the energy you expend will be equal to about 175 calories. The same time spent doing the JumpGa cardio element burns 205 calories – and it's much more fun!

## JUMPGA – PELVIC FLOOR SAVIOUR

Low-intensity, alternate Heel Bounce rebounding is a great choice to get your heart rate up without putting your pelvic floor at risk and will protect the pelvic floor. When the pelvic floor (the group of muscles and ligaments that surrounds and supports all the organs in the pelvis) is strong, it prevents problems such as incontinence. Working on a bungee trampoline has a lot of elasticity (softer bounce) to activate your muscles to bounce back up again. It works your pelvic floor and all the muscles recruiting more 'fast-twitch' fibres so you build up strength quickly.

Daily squeezing while you bounce will help keep the pelvic floor strong and can cure incontinence in 80 percent of cases. Women who haven't done this form of pelvic floor exercises before, and have leaking, will find that if they gently rebound a few times a day, in about two weeks they'll notice some difference. It's like any muscle: if you don't use it, you'll lose it.

## HOW TO DO THE HEEL BOUNCE

The Heel Bounce: stand on the rebounder with your feet about shoulder-width apart. Then gently lift alternate heels off the mat, just enough to cause your body to start bouncing very slightly. With each bounce, after lifting each heel off the mat a bit, gently press the opposite heel back into the mat. With a flat standing foot while you're doing this bounce technique: landing heel to toe, NOT toe to heel is the correct form. This ensures that your standing leg will receive the majority of your weight, which should be around 90 percent. Also, keep your knees slightly bent but not locked while bouncing. And when you're pushing your heels into the mat lift and contract your pelvic floor so it stays up for the duration to resist that downward pressure. Bouncing very gently in this way for about twenty minutes can provide you with huge health and wellness benefits.

## JUMPGA OUTPERFORMS SPINNING

During one of Wayne's guest-speaking appearances at Champney's a member of the audience asked him if he could prove that the cardio component of his JumpGa programme is really a high-performance work out. Another guest in the audience intervened before he could answer; saying that she could prove that his claims were really true. She introduced herself as a keen fitness fan and wearer of a 'Fitbit Blaze' (a health performance watch and app).

The activity tracker clearly showed that during the 20-minute cardio component of the JumpGa class that she attended, she had worked at her Peak Zone (high-intensity exercise zone) level longer than during the same time period in her Spinning class. As a result, other members have done the same and the results were similar; in that 20 minutes of JumpGa cardio does outperform a spinning class. It has not been scientifically tested but nevertheless, it all sounds promising. Strength doesn't come from what you can do, it comes from overcoming the things you once thought you couldn't do.

And finally… most gyms have a membership subscription that is more than ten times their capacity. This is a brilliant business model that succeeds when its customers don't set foot in the door but continue to pay their monthly membership fee to alleviate their guilt. Also classes are not for everyone: a survey found that 82% of gym members would prefer a home fitness plan. Just as there will be driverless cars, so health clubs will be digital spaces as well as 'bricks and mortar' places. Training at home is convenient, with no geographical barriers and without the customary pain strain or accompanying boredom. 'JUMPGA' is not about going to the gym three days a week to do the same routine over and over again. For the busy time-pushed non-exercisers the JUMPGA EXPRESS programmes are a total fitness workout in the shortest space of time: 4 to 10 minutes. It can be repeated (just like doing sets in weight training) – you choose how many sets you have time for, or how fit you are! It is something you can do on a daily basis and feel empowered, as you are improving your health. A rebounder is a proven fitness device that is sure to make anyone's day and life that much brighter and healthier. As long as you have enough room to hold a rebounder, you have space to train at home.

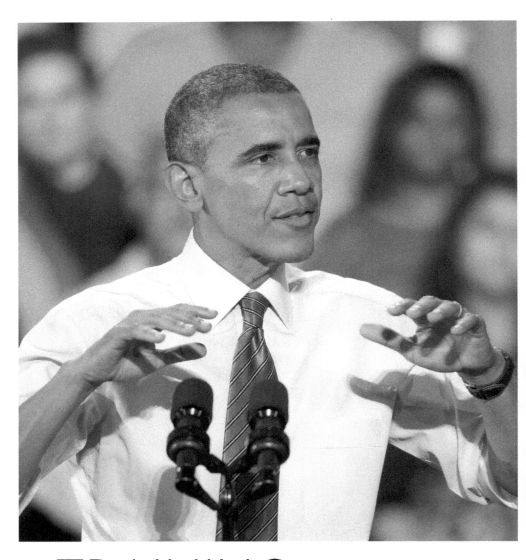

# TRAINING
# AND THE
# BUSINESS ELITE

# HUMAN PERFORMANCE IS OF CENTRAL IMPORTANCE

THE GREAT SCHOLAR Confucius considered human performance so important that he decreed 'if a man has reached forty or fifty without being heard of (acquired a good reputation through his performance in proper duties), he, indeed, is incapable of commanding respect.'

Eastern traditions offer support in the importance of human performance. Siddhartha Gautama the Buddha, who is widely misperceived, said that the right effort, the energetic will to perform rightly in the world, is one of the spokes of the central Eightfold Path. He maintained that one of the four keys to a layperson's happiness in life is excellent accomplishment born of persistent effort.

The world is full of amazing athletes and brilliant business men and women; but what divides the 'very good' from the world class? It's a willingness to do everything in their power to maximise their talent... that last little bit of effort sets them apart.

A proper training programme infiltrates every aspect of your life and helps improve your posture, exude more energy, and prepare you for how to handle the demands of a busy work-life schedule. Without the correct mindset you'll look and sound less authoritative in the office or compete less effectively out on the sports field. You can spot from a mile away the executive who exercises regularly – just from the way they look and how they radiate positivity, passion, vitality, and energy. The medal winners have a champion inside from the beginning of the event. Everyone experiences panic, be it in a competition or a top level meeting – success means overcoming it; structuring your belief system and achieving balance and self-confidence.

How we look, sound and communicate are the outward reflection of our mindset. For an athlete or top sportsman in a one-on-one competition, there is as much of a psychological battle as a physical one – convincing your opponent that you have the upper hand can go a long way towards tilting the fight in your favour. Equally believing in yourself, seeing yourself as the winner at the finishing line or the final whistle, will affect the game you play or how fast you run. This counts for captains of industry too – leaders must themselves adopt a positive mindset that will deliver a message to those around them. For CEOs in today's world, being fit isn't about health or vanity; it is an integral part of the job. If a top executive is visibly out of shape, he risks passing a message about his overall effectiveness and competence to those around him. Others in his immediate workplace are liable to perceive him as less effective in performance and in inter-personal relationships. In today's climate, exercise for top executives is no longer limited to forging deals out on the golf course.

*If exercise stops, then everything else will start falling apart. With the loss of physical health, productivity at work goes down.*

## THE HEALTH OF LEADERSHIP

Inherent in their position as business leaders, today's top executives tend to have wide-reaching responsibilities, carry a demanding work schedule and work ever longer hours in order to stay on top. Sadly their lifestyle is also filled with numerous pitfalls that can lead to chronic health conditions like diabetes, heart disease and high blood pressure. Typically the leaders of industry continue to personally invest incredible amounts of time to start, run and build a successful company, but are all too often unaware of the amount of stress their bodies are accumulating.

These leaders are at an increased risk of developing unseen health-related conditions, many of which could be easily prevented or corrected prior to stopping them from performing at the peak level required of their position.

The elite leaders among us undoubtedly possess a certain talent that distinguishes them from the rest of us mere mortals, but most also stand out as possessing self-confidence and a positive body image. Why are they devoted to health and exercise?

Entrepreneurs out there want to build something great, do something that matters and change the world. Business comes first and trumps everything else, family, friends and especially health: but it's a mistake. Exercise lifts up all other areas of your life – including business, so it must come first. As the entrepreneur, Joshua Steimle explains about his attitude to exercise, 'It makes me better in every role I have... husband, father, friend or entrepreneur. If I were to stop exercising because I felt that being a good business owner was a higher priority, then ironically I would end up a worse business owner than I was when it was a lower priority. Putting exercise first creates a win-win.'

The most successful people know they must mentally and physically push themselves. That's why many of them turn to intense exercise routines that push their boundaries, make them physically stronger, and improve their mental processing abilities. Studies have shown that staying physically active not only maintains general good health but can also prevent the onset of chronic diseases such as heart disease, osteoarthritis and dementia. A year-long study at the University of British Columbia involving ageing women and comparing the cognitive effects of different degrees of exercise found that among those who weight-trained there was an improvement not only in tests of memory and learning, but also in executive functions such as decision-making and conflict resolution.

The bottom line is that the truly successful leaders make time for daily exercise because they believe this will keep them ahead of the game. They have to prepare their bodies to handle the increasing demands of excessive hours and heavy travel schedules. Exercising gives them the focus, strength and endurance to communicate with energy throughout every day.

One of the keys to sticking at it is to do something you enjoy – hence captains of industry each have their own twist on how to keep fit.

Former US President Barack Obama is apparently 'not a morning person' – and yet he will wake up early to work out, using a combination

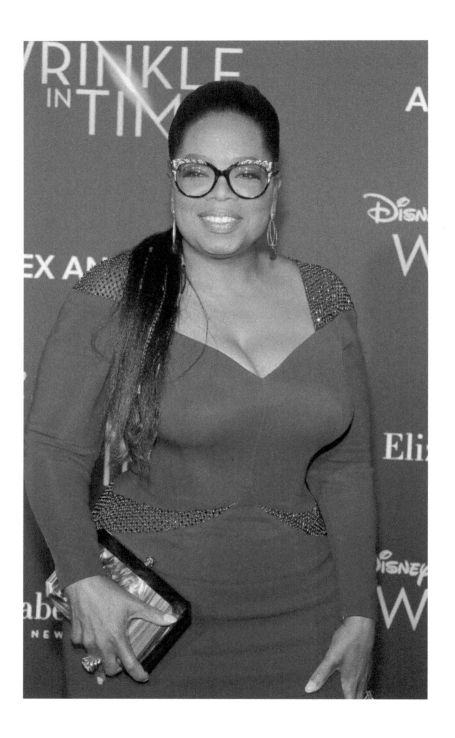

of strength and cardio training 45 minutes a day, six days a week. He admitted in his autobiography that he had been a casual drug user and under-achiever until he started running three miles a day. Now he sticks faithfully to his workout routine and has also been seen playing basketball around Washington.

TV star and one of the most powerful women in the world, Oprah Winfrey, trains hard to help her power through her busy days. Workouts with her trainer include 45 minutes of cardio six mornings a week and four to five strength training sessions per week including incline crunches and stretching. She also meditates, sitting in silence twice a day, for 20 minutes.

Richard Branson ranks as the only entrepreneur to have built eight separate billion dollar companies, not to mention being number 12 in the UK on Forbes' list of The World's Billionaires. He attributes some of his success to his energetic lifestyle and explains that 'Over my 50 years in business I have learned that if I rise early I can achieve so much more in a day, and therefore in life.' Waking at 5am gives him time he wouldn't normally have to exercise and spend time with his family before getting down to business. Richard's physical activities can include swimming, yoga, tennis, running and weight-lifting and he maintains that being fit and healthy, with the ensuing endorphin rush that comes from exercise, gives him four extra hours of productivity per day. Studies have repeatedly proven that exercise improves your mood by boosting your feel-good endorphins, but it can also make you more productive. Healthy physical activity improves mental capacity and lowers stress, which are both very important for a productive day.

Doctors to the billionaire Warren Buffet suggested a change of diet, but Warren loves his hamburgers, hot dogs and Coca Cola too much and instead opted for exercise as being the 'lesser of two evils'!

Anna Wintour, Editor in Chief of US Vogue, wakes at 5.45 every morning to be able to play tennis before her daily hair appointment and claims her routine keeps her 'disciplined and moving forward.'

Craig Esrael, CEO of First South Financial is now in his mid-50s and committed to fitness — his own and that of his employees. He was teased as an overweight child and young man, but turned his life around when he lost 65 pounds in one single summer. He now provides exercise programmes, healthy foods and a yoga class for managers, all in the workplace. For his own part, he gets up around 4am to walk and run around four miles, then does push-ups and sit-ups. Throughout the day he takes stairs rather than lifts, and uses push-up bars or weights whenever he has a spare moment. His exercise patterns are not dependent on location, or weather, or others; so he can maintain them anywhere and at any time. Versatility is of paramount importance for a frequently travelling CEO. As Craig points out, 'I may not be able to pack weights in my suitcase, but a jump rope and push-up bar fit just fine.'

**'Super-Ager is my go to fitness programme'**

Susan Rodway QC

Top CEOs are not only pushing themselves to exercise, but also working to institute health incentives in the workplace; understanding that if team members put exercise and health before their jobs, they might work fewer hours but they will feel better about themselves, have far more fulfilling lives and ultimately produce better results in the hours that they do work.

The simple answer to being more productive in business would seem to be to 'work out'. At the same time, though, it has to be what works best for each individual. In other words, you have to find the things; the workout, the activities that help you to achieve more, that make you more productive, and then make the time to accomplish those activities that will take you to higher levels.

**'I had a feeling of greater self-awareness after training with Wayne'**

Steven Greenhalgh,
Former Deputy Mayor of London

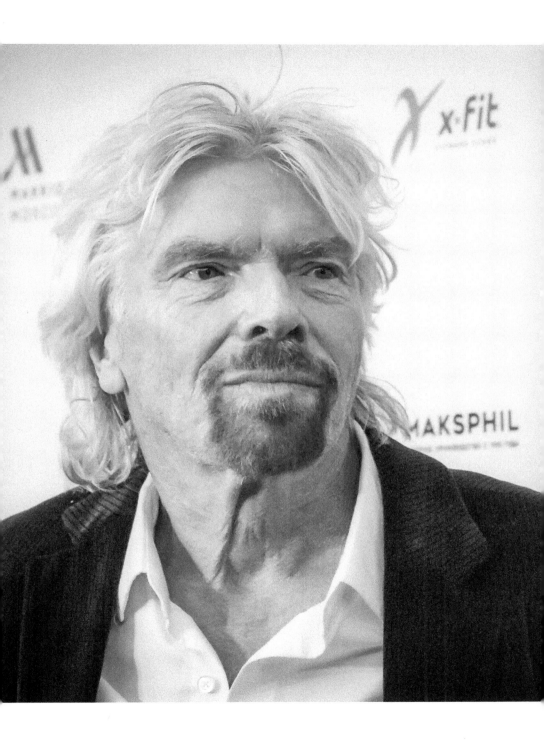

## LEADERS – WHETHER MALE OR FEMALE – NEED A BALANCED BODY AND MIND

Most people who do exercise have relatively fixed training routines – often decreed by what they have always done for years. If there was one form of exercise that I believe more captains of industry should participate in it would be yoga. But first they will need to ditch the old-school mentality that yoga is for women.

I started yoga twenty years ago, at a time when supposedly real men did not do yoga. We were given toys (i.e. weights) to play with and told that that's the manly way to exercise and occupy your mind.

The commonly perpetuated 'yoga myths' – that yoga isn't a decent workout, that you have to be flexible to do it, that men's bodies just aren't built for yoga poses – are in part true, but not at the core of the reason why men don't do it. The answer has been there for years – social conditioning telling us that to be a man we had to look and behave a certain way, when we don't. This is why the vast majority of Western men will automatically walk into a weights room but have never turned to yoga as a way of exercise.

There is no hard wiring at birth, it is society's expectations that are at the root of behavioural differences between men and women. All men have learned behaviour of how people assume they will be. We are expected and encouraged to be strong at sport and have the ability to fix things. Every trait that we have is moulded by experience. For lots of guys I know there are aspects of yoga that can be a turnoff, but when it's explained in a way that is understandable to them, they don't have a problem with concepts like empathy or expressing their emotions.

The yoga community is heavily female-dominated as a consequence of a self-fulfilling prophecy that yoga is for women, largely perpetuated by the media surrounding the health industry itself. According to Yoga Alliance Professionals there are 300 million yoga practitioners in the world, of which it is estimated that 75% are female.

It is a billion dollar market and also the 4th-fastest growing industry in the USA. The amount of money spent by yoga practitioners has risen by 87% in the last five years. Yes, perhaps the sound-bites are saying that more men should take up yoga, but not loudly enough to upset the apple cart.

If you've attended a yoga class recently, the chances are that a good portion of practitioners, if not all of them, will be women. Mainstream media yoga magazines, newspapers et al, all use images of beautiful, slender, taut woman to sell their products. So, unsurprisingly, a lot of men have become socially conditioned to see yoga as an unmanly, female domain, the bottom line being that it is something their girlfriend or wife does, but they won't.

Generally, men spend a lot of time in their heads, making them very disconnected from their bodies. When they do exercise it usually has a competitive edge, unnecessarily pushing their bodies to their limit. Yoga asana encourages men to give themselves permission to slow down and to learn how to focus their breath in a meaningful way, one that joins all the bits of them together for a balanced body and mind.

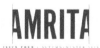

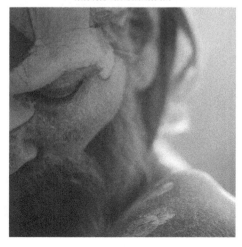

A progressive magazine that has pioneered new types of feature writing in Yoga journalism

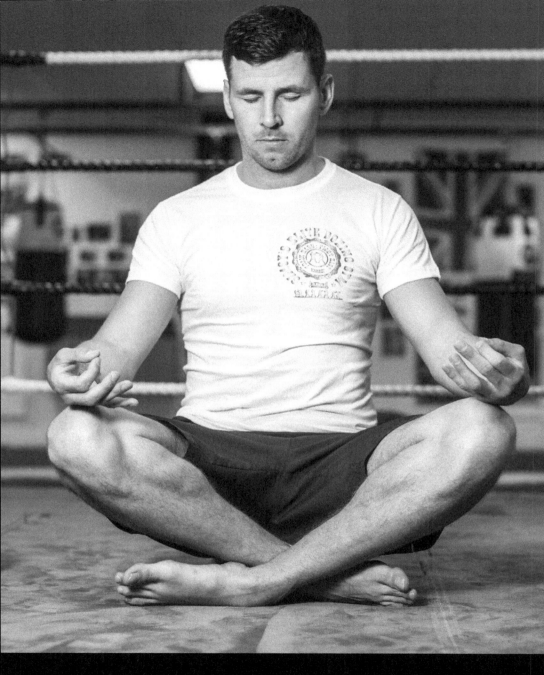

# TRAINING THE
# SPORTING ELITE

# THE BOXER'S JOURNEY:
# NURTURING THE CHAMPION'S WILL

IT'S A STRANGE thing. When you look at Wayne's life, although it shares with most of us a fair number of ups and downs, there is something very consistent about how Wayne always seems to seize the moment and manage to be in the right place at the right time. He says, 'It's when preparation meets opportunity'. What were the odds of Darren Barker, the boxer from Barnet, crossing paths with Wayne Lèal, non-boxing Fulham boy? Pretty remote, one would have thought, but it did happen. It turned out they were both staunch Chelsea fans who just happened to go to the same fitness club on the Chelsea football stadium site. Neither one knew about the other. Darren would go to the gym to lift weights, whilst Wayne never went to the gym but was always in the swimming pool. Then one fateful day they did speak, and it proved to be the beginning of a most successful partnership.

At the end of one of Darren's training sessions, Wayne was sitting in the lounge area, drinking a protein shake after his workout, when Darren walked by. Out of the blue, Wayne asked, 'How was your session?' Darren replied, 'Okay I guess,' to which Wayne said, 'Why don't you sit down and let's talk about how we can change that?' Darren, somewhat surprised by Wayne's offer, did take a seat, intrigued as to what Wayne might have to say to him. We often hear about people getting a sense of déjà vu, as if they have met in a previous life. If there was ever any truth behind this, Darren and Wayne were a great example. Here were two people who had never met before, turning a brief chat into an hour-long conversation and feeling like two friends who had known each other for ever. Darren told Wayne that he had seen him training in the pool and was intrigued that Wayne not only looked great but that he trained so differently to the other guys in the gym – avoiding the run-of-the-mill cardio and weightlifting. At the end of their conversation, Wayne invited Darren to join him in one of his pool sessions and Darren, with his interest piqued, immediately agreed.

Wayne's programme was created with a slightly older generation in mind, but it has been tried and endorsed by an increasing number of younger fitness seekers. Darren Barker was about to join their ranks.

If Darren were placed in the Trans-theoretical Model (TTM) at the time of his meeting with Wayne, he would be at the 'pre-contemplation' stage. He was in automatic mode, not realising that he was just going through the motions with his usual training regime: a routine of treadmill running, weight training and sit-ups – and didn't acknowledge that a drastic change was needed. At that moment he had very little prospect of any fights, hence he was training only to keep fit rather than for an upcoming challenge.

Even though he was not fighting fit, Darren felt confident that he could handle any training that Wayne could throw at him and that he would be fitter than Wayne, who was much older and had never competed professionally. Darren went to a pool session (Kun-Aqua) with an air of confidence, imagining that it would be a fairly easy workout. As a result, Wayne's warning at the beginning of the session re the deceptive nature of the exercises went unheeded. Wayne says that every guy he teaches does the same thing: 'They become driven by their ego to be better and fitter than me, even though I'm the one who created the damn thing, kind of funny isn't it? I have seen this happen on every occasion!' Before the session ended, Darren said, 'I'm f••••d mate, how much more of this is there?' He, like everyone, was surprised by the degree to which the resistance of the water magnified the level of energy required for each movement. Needless to say, Darren did not make it to the end of the pool session and Wayne even had to tone down the session to account for Darren's lack of fitness.

Darren was now on his way to being converted to the Super-Ager programme, but his induction was not quite complete, as he still had the JumpGa to try. This was as much of a surprise and challenge to him as the Kun-Aqua workout. Again, Darren was left gasping for air and discovering that he was really out of condition and as inflexible as a lamppost. Darren had now experienced for himself the exercise regimes involved in the Super-Ager programme. The absence of any immediate prospect of a fight did not motivate him to take a new direction in his training, but it certainly gave him a lot of food for thought. They continued to bump into each other in the club on a regular basis, but the relationship was different. Darren now had a greater respect for Wayne and his methodology, having experienced the training for himself.

A few weeks later Darren called Wayne to tell him that Eddie Hearn, his promoter, had a possible title elimination fight for him and that he wanted Wayne to be his strength and conditioning coach. After saying yes, Wayne, who is not a religious man, came off the phone to Darren, rolled his eyes up to the sky and said, 'Thank you, God.' Wayne believed that this was the opportunity that he had waited for all of his life – to take what he does to another level, knowing that although he was not actually in the ring himself his protégé would be.

There were plenty of twists and turns to follow, as two weeks later the distinct possibility of a title fight appeared. Daniel Geale was defending his IBF World Middleweight Title and chose Darren Barker as his opponent – possibly thinking him to be a relatively soft touch because in his previous world title challenge he had been stopped by Sergio Martinez in Atlantic City by a knockout in the eleventh round.

Darren told Wayne about his previous injuries and hip surgery that had left him inactive for over a year. The bottom line was that Darren was incapable of doing the traditional boxing training: morning runs, skipping, weightlifting and sit-ups because they left him in constant pain during and after training. For Wayne Lèal this was exciting but scary, yet at the same time, he knew that he had the distinct advantage of empathy – having suffered similar injuries himself and developed a strategy of managing and moving through the pain.

It has to be mentioned what a leap of faith Darren was taking; having only met Wayne a few weeks previously and entrusting him with the biggest opportunity of his life. Wayne's training methodology would go against the grain of all boxing premise and there was the possibility of him becoming a laughing stock. Twitter comments were plentiful: 'Are you going to start eating mung beans, Darren?' 'Will you wear Jesus sandals into the ring?' 'Are you going to 'OM' before the fight?' What Darren was doing wasn't considered to be very manly.

He did however capture the imagination of sports writers around the world, including a double page spread in *The Times* newspaper with the headline 'Boxer Darren Barker takes up yoga for title fight' and the tongue-in-cheek introduction: 'This middleweight thinks warrior pose can help him win the world title. It's not exactly Rocky Balboa,' wrote journalist Robert Crampton. Despite the cynicism, Darren was undeterred. He was dedicated and followed the regime. In committing to Wayne's somewhat alternative form of training, he was 'working' long hours: spending 1.5 to 2 hours of daily training with Wayne, followed by 2 hours in the ring every afternoon. Yet there he was at 6.30am, sitting outside Wayne's Fulham studio, ready and waiting.

The sessions were initially divided between physical and mental exercise, or sometimes they spent time simply talking – about where Darren was in his career and where he really wanted to get to.

During one of these talks, Darren revealed something that he had never told anyone: when he fought for the world title against Sergio Martinez, he didn't actually believe that he could win. This crucial secret told Wayne a lot about his mental attitude and gave him a direction to follow. Darren embraced all aspects of his new training – taking to it with absolute commitment.

It was clear from the beginning that Darren had never really had a mind and body training strategy; he would just work out with a personal trainer, doing what he had always done because he didn't know any different way. He said that the first thing that became very apparent when he trained with Wayne for the sample sessions was that – unlike his previous physical exercises, that led to pain not gain – this time he was injury free during and after the workout.

During the first official session, Wayne asked Darren, 'If you were the World Champion now, how would you sit?' Unknowingly Darren immediately sat up straighter, adopting a position of greater presence, and it was from this moment that Darren knew Wayne was the real deal and he'd arrived at the right place at the right time in his life. His goal was to be World Champion and he placed his trust in Wayne as his mentor, as someone offering a path that could get him there. By the third session, he was hooked and, with this established, their strategy was defined.

In every exercise regime you need strength, resistance and flexibility. But for a boxer at Darren's level, control is hugely important, to increase his mental focus, to be cool under pressure. Darren said, 'At the end of the week, I'm more focused and my abdominals hurt without having done a single sit up. As for all the other stuff, I reckon I've found something that isn't just a replacement for the old-school approach, but something that is actually better.'

For the next 12 weeks of training, they followed an agreed routine – dividing time between pool work, the rebounder, and yoga (the three disciplines of Super-Ager). Each routine was followed by a guided visualisation session of 5 to 10 minutes. In his head, Darren became a champion before achieving the actual title – and once the clear goal was established, the mental process of talking and behaving like a champion gave him the essential level of confidence and determination.

Wayne said that when he works with clients, he tries to find out as much as he can about the individual. Something seemingly unimportant can be the little gem that makes the biggest difference to the outcome. During one of the sessions, Darren talked about different influences in his life, such as his mother's love for R&B. He said she would play it constantly, to the point where he even listens to it himself. Wayne said, 'This was a nugget of information that I used. Darren really loved his Mum, so I would play R&B music during our training sessions – using yet another sense and invoking positive memories to reinforce current action. It was also fun. Training has to be fun, otherwise, motivation becomes an additional, unnecessary challenge.'

A strategy will always remain just a strategy unless it has a trigger – something that a lot of people are not fully aware of unless involved in a competitive sporting activity. It's the trigger that puts someone in competition mode, into that state of readiness, standing a chance of success. It may be a starting gun, a referee's whistle or, in Darren's case, the referee's bell. When he is sparring there is the bell, and when he was doing circuits with Wayne there was always a bell at the beginning, and at the end, of his interval training.

Wayne is a Master NLP (Neuro-Linguistic Programming) practitioner, and all of Darren's sessions incorporated guided meditation. Whether Darren was lying on a yoga mat, sitting on the sofa or floating on his back in the pool – Wayne always made time for at least 5 minutes of meditation. Wayne incorporated four crucial elements of NLP:

- Visualisation – Barker used visualisation techniques, created by Wayne, to help him see, think and feel like a World Middleweight Champion. Wayne had Barker engage in visualisation as part of his training ritual, turning Barker's brain into a virtual film of his imminent success.

- Affirmations – affirmations, like the visualisations, were another part of Wayne's mind-reprogramming technique. Wayne had Barker repeat various affirmations that were linked to his goals. He recited phrases such as: 'Real strength is about conditioning the mind to think confidently.' 'I will, I can, I'm going to.' After every training session, Wayne would feed Darren's mind with statements about how power is not only measured in terms of what you have but also what your opponent thinks you have.

- Mistakes can always teach us something new – Wayne told Barker that the best lessons come from being defeated; that's the place where the hardest but truest lessons are learned.

- Goals – together, Wayne and Darren set the goal of Darren becoming the middleweight champion of the world. Wayne told him, 'You are in charge of your mind; therefore, the outcome of the fight is up to you; and losing is not an option. The boxer with greater belief, desire, and intelligence is always the one who wins.'

In the following weeks, Darren began to talk and behave more and more like a champion. His belief in himself had been renewed. He could picture himself lifting the title belt high and totally believed in what he was doing with Wayne.

Wayne wasn't part of Darren's inner circle of friends, including his manager and boxing trainer Tony Simms. Wayne did travel to the fight in Atlantic City – but he paid for his own flight and hotel for himself and his son. In a sense, he had as much riding on the outcome as Darren himself. Darren traditionally spoke to no one, outside his inner circle, in the build-up to a big fight – concentrating his mind and energy. The weigh-in was the first time Wayne had witnessed the atmosphere of a major boxing event, and he found it electric, with the British fans who'd followed Darren across the Atlantic making their voices heard. Darren looked confident and relaxed.

A few hours before the fight Wayne was surprised to receive a message saying that Darren wanted to see him. Wayne had no idea what Darren wanted and when he got to the suite, Darren's ex-wife Gemma opened the door, said, 'He's in the bedroom waiting to see you' and left. When Wayne entered, Darren said, 'Mate, I'm nervous, my confidence is not there.' Darren had turned to Wayne for help in lifting him up again. He continued, 'I don't know what's come over me, but I feel really nervous and I just needed to talk to you. Can you help me?' This conveyed an enormous responsibility and was a pivotal moment – trusting Wayne and admitting a weakness at this stage, rather than turning to his inner circle for help. Getting him relaxed and focused was essential. Wayne had to think on his feet, there was a worldwide audience waiting to see if Darren could pull off a momentous victory, and it was imperative that Darren saw the victory as the only conceivable outcome. So, he sat Darren in a chair by the window of his hotel room, looking out over Atlantic City, and told him to close his eyes and concentrate on his breathing putting Darren into a state of hypnosis. He began to speak, using the analogy of a book, telling Darren, 'I am a publisher and I am commissioning you to write your story about becoming the World Middleweight Champion: it can be a short story: one chapter, or an epic tale: twelve chapters.' Wayne's carefully chosen words set Darren visualising different scenarios of the fight going the twelve-round distance or lasting just one round. Either way, he was going to be the new champion, because this book was about the success that Wayne had already planted in his mind. This final visualisation session between Wayne and Darren reinstated Darren's mental belief that he could and would win.

While Darren's eyes were closed, he began to slip into a deep, relaxed hypnotic state. Wayne talked about throwing punches and could see Darren's body twitching with every punch he threw: a head movement to slip a jab, throwing a hook followed by an uppercut, his hands clenching or relaxing in tune with Wayne's words.

Wayne's final suggestion was to end the book with the voice of the famous ring commentator, Michael Buffer, delivering the memorable line '…and the new World Middleweight title holder is…' This was something that Darren always mentioned when they were training together so Wayne made it his ultimate symbol of victory. This book was his action metaphor, to leave behind all the things that were holding him back. When the session finished Darren opened his eyes and sat in silence for a while with a 'winner's smile' on his face, then said, 'Thank you, I feel much better now.' Wayne told him not to say any more and left the room silently.

In Darren's relaxed state, Wayne had told him to stop fighting his feelings of self-doubt and never being quite good enough, but rather to accept them as something everyone has sometimes. He got Darren to concentrate on the belief that there are no limits because everything is possible; and right there, right then, was his moment of power. He basically helped Darren to rewire his own beliefs and thoughts about himself and reinstate his winning mentality.

What Wayne did worked because the training sessions aligned Darren's physical strength with his mental belief. The bottom line was that both boxers trained hard to be in the ring that day; the deciding factor was who truly wanted it more.

In the now famous sixth round, Darren went down to a massive body shot from Geale, but picked himself up from the canvas on the

*Darren Barker became the first boxer in modern history to become a World Champion without doing the traditional running, skipping, sit-ups or weight lifting.*

count of nine. He had an inner belief that could not accept defeat; and of course, his core strength training made a difference in enabling him to withstand such a body shot. At that moment, Wayne knew the outcome; the fight went the distance. It was now down to the judges' scorecards and when Michael Buffer, said; 'And the new World Middleweight title holder is Darren Barker,' there was pandemonium everywhere. When Darren lifted the title belt, it was the ultimate confirmation for Wayne that his training programme worked. He had become part of the elite group of coaches that has trained a champion.

Following the victory, a media frenzy began: everyone wanted a piece of Darren Barker now that he had reached celebrity status. There was an endless list of functions and invites to prestigious events, like the men's' GQ awards. Darren was in demand. There was only a relatively short space of time before the next fight: against the German Champion Felix Sturm. Surprisingly this fight took place abroad, in Germany. It was unusual for a defending champion to fight his first title defence abroad, but Darren accepted it because the money on the table was too good to be refused.

Wayne said that the training between the Geale and Sturm training camps was markedly different. Darren, perhaps feeling over-confident, did not adhere to their training programme as rigorously as he had previously done.

Darren was sure that he would have no problem beating Felix Sturm: but it wasn't quite so clear-cut and he had a totally different demeanour.

There were a number of missed training sessions due to his social and promotional appointments. Pool training is a major component of Wayne's training regime and for reasons beyond their control, it never happened in the preparation for the Sturm fight. Over the coming weeks, they even had to tone down the intensity of their rebounding and yoga sessions because Darren picked up niggling injuries while sparring in the ring.

Wayne wanted Darren to use an NLP technique called 'Pattern Interrupt'. In this instance, it would have involved buying Darren time in the ring by giving Sturm something to think about: introducing an element that he hadn't planned for and throwing him off his game. Wayne said to Darren: 'Sturm probably lives and breathes videos of you and knows you for your distinctive hairstyle. What do you think will happen if you change your appearance at the last minute before entering the arena? – shave your head completely, for instance! Enter the ring with a hood and then, when you pull off your hood; Sturm, the crowd, and even the commentators are going to think w.t.f. (what the f••k)!' Darren laughed and said he'd think about it.

On the afternoon of the fight, Wayne received a call from a friend, Charlie – a professional gambler. Charlie asked whether he should place a hefty £25,000 bet on Darren to win. Wayne said, 'Give me a few minutes,' then immediately called Darren and asked how he was feeling. Darren said he felt good, but when Wayne asked if he planned to do what they had discussed (i.e. to shave his head), Darren laughed and replied, 'No, not a chance mate!' Wayne called Charlie back straightaway and told him to keep his money in his pocket.

When Felix dropped Darren to the canvas twice in the second round Wayne said that his heart sank; because there was nothing he could do to help. When Darren turned to the corner pointing to his hip, Wayne immediately knew that he wouldn't be able to continue – and soon afterward his corner threw in the towel.

Wayne believed that the absence of pool training contributed to Darren's inability to maintain his previous level of physical intensity. The pool training programme had worked on improving his core stabilisation and mobility in the ring. He felt that Darren's muscle stabilisation was compromised; so that this became an issue of stability versus mobility—each attribute inevitably comes at the expense of the other so that each joint had to make a trade-off between structural sturdiness and manoeuvrability.

The hip joint has immense structural stability for weight-bearing purposes, and the pool training was crucial to maintaining the mobility of his hip joint for spine and core stability. Hence the loss to Felix may have been inevitable because Darren's movement and stability were compromised.

After that fight, Darren made the decision to retire from boxing – but just think what a legacy he has left behind. He was the first boxer in modern history to achieve world championship status without running, skipping, sit-ups or weight training. From being a 12-year-old boy setting out on a journey, he had arrived at Wayne's training studio – and taken the brave decision to follow a different physical conditioning programme, one that won him a world championship title.

Darren had the last laugh... reporters scoffed at his change of mental and physical tactics beforehand, but he has the belt to prove that it worked. He followed his dream and made it come true. Wayne's final prediction to Darren all those years ago was that he should be a television boxing pundit. Darren said I don't have the confidence... 'I can be my own worst enemy.' But fast forward three years and just as Wayne predicted Darren can now be seen regularly on television as a boxing pundit, with nearly ninety thousand followers on Twitter hanging onto his every word.

And finally... Wayne responded to *Times* reporter Robert Crampton's claim that Darren was delusional; 'If Barker has discovered the holy grail of physical conditioning, stamina, and strength without having to run or lift weights, he will be a very popular man indeed'. Well guess what Robert, he WON.

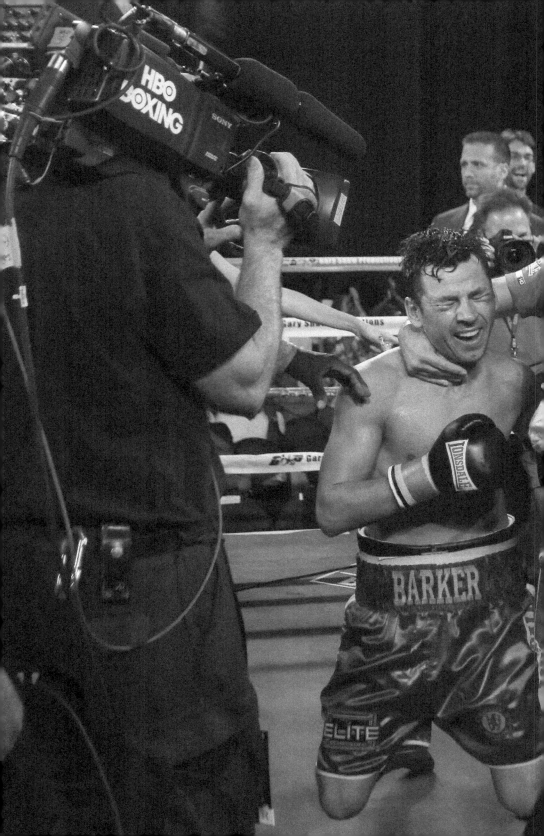

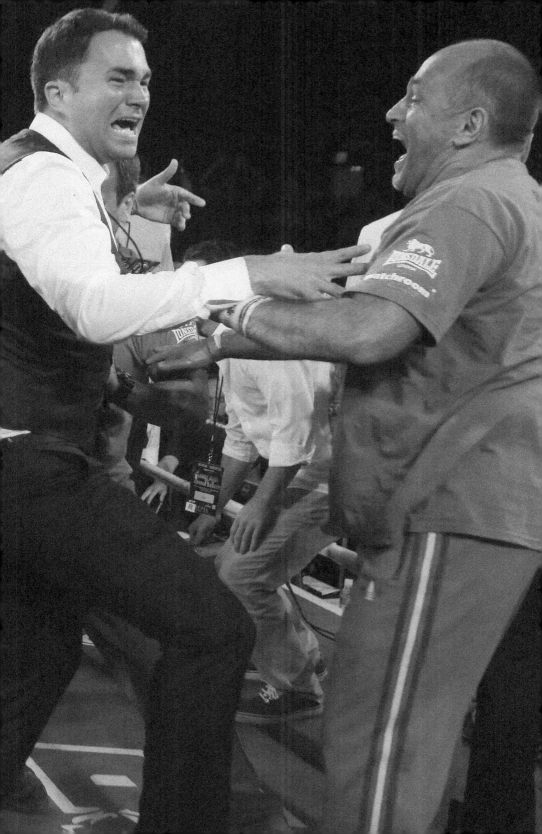

# RYAN BERTRAND –
# TAKING IT TO THE NEXT LEVEL

Athletes and sportsmen of calibre tend to have relatively fixed training routines – often decreed by their manager, the club they play for, or the specifics of their chosen sport.

Sometimes, though, physical problems, or a specific injury will necessitate a change in training. Sometimes the athlete needs an extra push or an alternative route to get to their goal. In some cases, they may even have lost sight of their goal and need a new training style, a new trigger to set them back on course and into the right space for a particular competition. Super-Ager fitness is a resistance-based programme – intensive yet without placing excessive strain on muscles or joints. It can be beneficial as a replacement or a complement to an athlete's more habitual or traditional training methods, regardless of the specific sport – it can work for tennis stars or boxers, gymnasts or footballers or javelin throwers.

## WORTH A GO

Back in 2012, Ryan Bertrand was playing left back for Chelsea as understudy to Ashley Cole. He'd heard about Darren Barker's success in the boxing ring after training with Wayne Lèal and came to him wanting to try out the technique for himself, hoping it would also work on the football pitch. Wayne said, 'Success comes to those who want it more. I could see in Ryan his hunger to succeed and his willingness to do anything to achieve his goal'. Ryan was a successful young footballer (23 years old at the time), earning thousands, living an enviable lifestyle and training in a state of the art complex – but nevertheless lacking belief in his own ability and turning to Wayne for help.

He came looking for a mentor – someone to give him that extra confidence in himself. Despite his status with a top club, Ryan had started asking himself who he was, what he wanted and where he was going in life. He admits that a large part of the game is a psychological battle. What comes into play is the character of the athlete and what one player is willing to do that another player is not. It's that last little bit of effort that separates them.

Wayne's exercise studio was in a Fulham street next door to a painter and decorator – who, whilst a friend of Wayne's, nevertheless found Ryan's appearance at the studio incredible: 'It's a joke: he has a state of the art complex and he's coming to your tiny s…hole of a studio to train!'

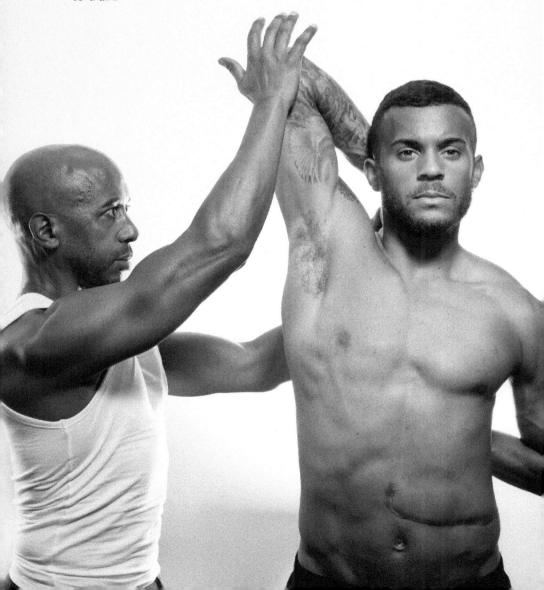

There he was though, in need of a new incentive and something original and different to build up his confidence. 'It's raised a few eyebrows in the changing room,' he admitted. 'I was looking to increase my speed, strength and explosiveness…In football it's all about short sharp bursts enabling me to get from A to B as quickly as possible.' Training on the rebounder is all about intense repetitions of short sequences of exercises – a common link already!

Ryan Bertrand's trust in Wayne was built up through actually seeing a physical change in himself and feeling a change in his attitude. Adopting Wayne's training regime he experienced an increase in his speed, strength and reactions, but also acknowledged the psychological benefits of the training methodology. 'At the beginning of each session, we just talk. We discuss the game, but also events outside of football, things happening in life that also affect performance. Voicing problems before a punishing work-out can be a release. You kind of reset and recharge.'

Wayne believes that a professional is someone who can do what needs to be done no matter how he feels within. Most footballers are just footballers in their attitude emotionally. A Premier League footballer must be different in the way he thinks and feels – and it is this ability to perform under the most trying conditions that separates out an elite performer.

In contrast to Darren Barker's training period – which was a clear 12-week period before his title fight – Ryan Bertrand's training was very focused and to be completed 'as soon as possible'. He wanted change and results and he wanted them 'now'.

During his training sessions with Wayne he also voiced frustrations. Wayne told him not to smile at his opponent because it's a sign of weakness: 'Look at your opponent like you want to run through him not past him'. In any team it is necessary to prove oneself, and he saw part of his problem as being his general 'Mr Nice Guy' image. On the pitch it's essential to generate a more aggressive persona: 'You have to present a façade… You get the sense that it's a battle that can be harder for players with a naturally more easy-going disposition. '

Wayne knew that Ryan needed more than an improvement in his football to get back into first team contention for club and country. He needed public exposure, and Wayne made it possible for Ryan to appear on BBC's *Football Focus* show – exceptional since only a certain number of players were offered a slot on the programme each season, and Ryan was not in Chelsea's first team. In conjunction with this *The Times* newspaper wanted to do an article on him and his training programme with Wayne. Ryan was, of course, excited at this prospect – but he was discouraged from appearing (a decision he bitterly regretted) by his management team. Since Ryan was not in the first team, it would have looked bad for Chelsea Football Club if he were chosen over other team members to appear on the stellar football show.

In the end, by way of a compromise, Ryan did the *Times* interview, featuring his training with Wayne, but the CFC (Chelsea Football Club) press officer was there and fielding questions – as might be expected. The answer to the question 'Who was your most influential manager?' slipped out uncensored though: Brendan Rogers, now manager at Celtic! The press officer almost choked on his cup of tea, probably wondering what Jose Mourinho, the then Chelsea manager, would say when he saw Ryan's answer.

At the beginning of 2015, Ryan transferred to Southampton and Wayne hasn't heard from him since. The story doesn't end there though. Wayne entered into discussions regarding the training of Darryll Williams; the former English Super Middleweight champion.

Darryll already knew about Wayne's success with Darren Barker but what he didn't know about was his work with Ryan; and Wayne coaching Ryan's 'nice guy on the pitch' image out of him. Wayne had told Ryan, 'look into your opponent's eyes and, without words, let your expression communicate "I'm not going to run around you, but through you"'. On hearing this Darryll laughed, saying; 'I met Ryan recently; and that was exactly what he told me he does when going onto the pitch.'

Bullet-proof evidence reinforcing the success of Wayne's influence! Ryan may not have stayed in touch, but he obviously never forgot what Wayne said – or how he made him feel.

…And so, Wayne's words continue to be passed on through Darren, Ryan and countless others.

Ryan's story also featured in an article in *The Times* January 14, 2014: 'Ryan Bertrand: trampolining keeps me super fit', by Ben Machell.

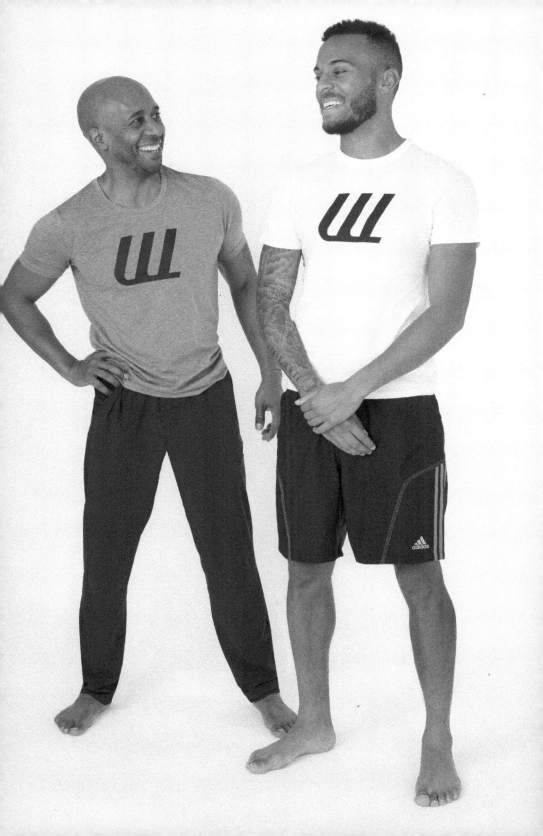

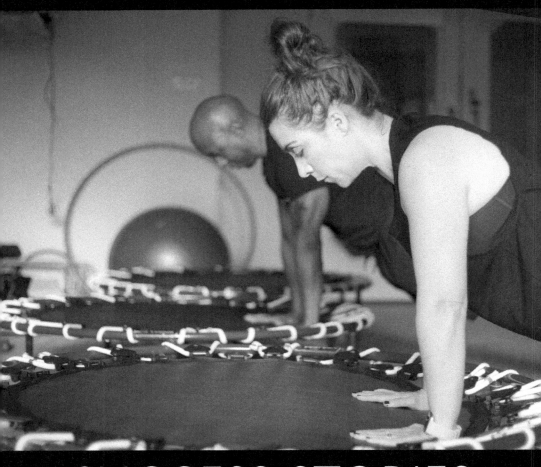

# SUCCESS STORIES – SPAS, INJURIES AND JOURNEYS TO HEALTH

# SANUS PER AQUAM

WAYNE HAS BEEN going to Champneys in Tring as a guest speaker, trainer and health coach for some time now. The exotic health spas of the Far East or even the Mediterranean offer more glitz, glamour and a good deal more sunshine – but Champneys he says, is the epitome of Englishness and all the more delightful for it.

Having worked at a number of the world's top spas Wayne recognises that the spa world is an evolving business and spa travellers are more clued up. He says: 'Retreats like my SUPER-AGER Fitness will be a bigger trend because people are more aware of their health and spas play a big part in that. No longer is it just the aesthetic massage, hair, nails, etc. Spas have to be seen to be giving a meaningful contribution to our mental and physical health.'

Most spas are the domain of middle-class women with time and money. So, Champneys has taken a bold move to make it more accessible to everyone by opening their doors to a wider audience: spa days, spa breaks, hen group getaways, romantic mini-breaks, to even advertising on male-dominated platforms.

There have been so many changes in the fitness industry over the past few years – the rise of extreme sports, extreme workouts, frantic exercise sessions fitted around busy work and social schedules, fads and fashions that work and others that don't. Places like Champneys have trainers, therapists and medical staff on hand who can analyse everything from food sensitivity screening to your DNA if you want a full health check! Or if you so choose, you can 'sweat your ass off' with bikes, boot camps and tennis. With so many options, you assume every class is full. There are lists and leaflets detailing what's on offer, but it seems there is only so much to be done in persuading people to have fun or to initiate a change in themselves. The old saying 'you can lead a horse to water...' is oh so true! You would think that the chance to try something new or at least to learn about it, no strings attached, would have a certain appeal –

but Wayne comments on a sad tendency towards apathy, with the gym and pool underused for much of every day.

As Wayne comments, 'Spas in general offer it all, but they can't drag their clients round and sit them in a class or drop them into the pool. The majority of guest go to be pampered rather than to improve!'

Despite this, Wayne's SUPER-AGER Fitness talks are among the best attended of all talks at the spa. His empathy for his clients is an element of his talks and workshops that has drawn many a reluctant convert. For an audience it means a lot to see him acting and reacting to them, rather than simply delivering a lecture. Everything that he is teaching in his programme, he has discovered for himself. Public speaking in itself is an art form and speaking from experience about a subject you have personally tried and tested gives an extra edge to your talk. Wayne is an example as well as an instructor: 'Do what I say AND what I do'. Living something yourself and then passing on personal experiences gives the listener so much more confidence in the validity of the advice.

The ladies at Champneys like Wayne – and the men too, but the ladies feel safe, pampered, understood. 'He doesn't shout at you like some personal trainers do...'. The audience at weekly talks does vary, with no stereotypical attendee: he may be speaking to women on outings together, dedicated ladies alone and partners tagging along; the lady in the street or the TV star taking a break. Wayne has looked out at his audience and seen famous faces smiling back – all warrant the same attention, the same degree of infectious enthusiasm and energy.

There isn't a set script – the talk varies depending on the audience and what they present: both in terms of inspiration and challenge. He has met the know-it-alls – regular visitors to health spas, who have done the treatments, seen the film and know everything there is to know about gyms and spas and, well just about everything – and still managed to tell them a thing or two! He has listened patiently to the belligerent lady: 'Why is this going to work for me? I've tried everything, done gyms and therapies – they can't fix me' – and proven her wrong. He has comforted the tearful soul who related stories of illness or loss and cried bitterly, embarrassing herself but not phasing him, and found positive words to reassure her. He has steered the conversation skilfully away from the lady in the front row who tried to take over the talk, who had a problem for every statement, an ailment for every occasion, and thought hers were of far more interest than anyone else's. Yet he still worked her examples into his talks and let her leave feeling important and 'noticed'.

Feedback collected on forms after the talks is consistently full of compliments and phrases such as 'very relaxed and motivational', 'natural', 'brilliant', 'I have already started to action his recommendations', 'I wish I had found his class years ago'...

Visitors to Champneys can be 'classified' according to the Transtheoretical Model on which Wayne based his SUPER-AGER Fitness – identifying where they are in a fitness programme or their process of self-discovery.

At his retreats he explains how and why each exercise will benefit you and help you rewire your own beliefs and thoughts about yourself. He enables you to see where you are, to develop your goal and the essential attitude needed to start making changes towards making your life physically and mentally better. Having such a programme that works on producing measurable results against a specific positive goal gives constant feedback and incentive to keep going. When your health starts to fail it overshadows everything else. Making a commitment; re-evaluating your life and taking on healthier habits will have a far-reaching payoff – you will feel better in everything you do.

Each person takes away a different aspect of SUPER-AGER Fitness when they leave. Some may opt to follow it as a stand-alone programme, others incorporate aspects of it into their exercise routines and their lives, often attracted by its low impact but high effect. Cathy is one of many regular visitors to Champneys. Already fit, but interested in exercise per se, she was intrigued and then enthused by Wayne's SUPER-AGER Fitness: 'It was exciting to find I could get the same results I'd achieved elsewhere in a much less stressful, more sustainable and ultimately fun way. I even occasionally remember to be more mindful: even if it's literally stopping on my bike to see, smell and listen to the forest on a remote road in Corsica, to savour the specific taste of the food I put in my mouth or just smiling from ear to ear remembering something or someone who gave me intense pleasure.'

Wayne has hosted workshops around the world – he says: 'In places like Thailand and Bali there is a stronger emphasis on eco-travel and environmental awareness of their treatments to the functionality of their facilities. Yet you can see the original Champneys concept in all the World's top spas.'

**Wayne with Paul Stainthorpe the UK's No 1 men's fitness blogger**

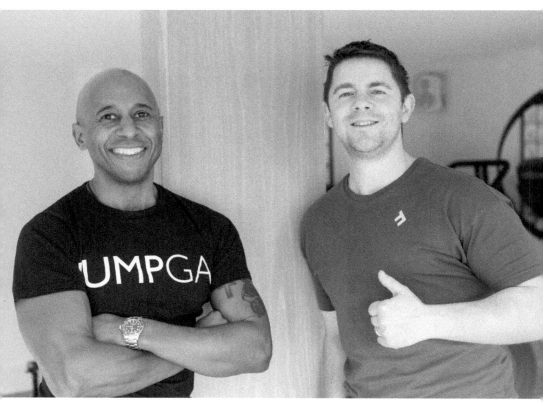

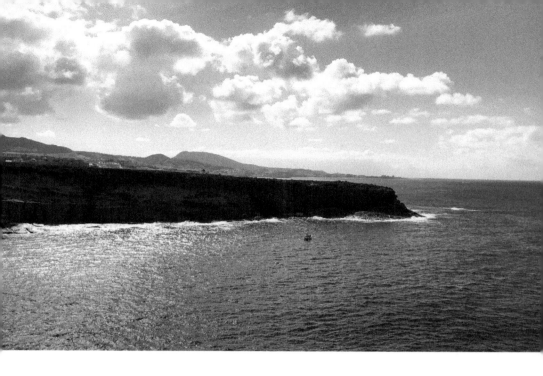

# HELEN SUTTON – NEW BEGINNINGS

I'm not a frequent visitor to health spas, although I have used the spa facilities in quite a few hotels around the world during my travels – the sauna, the massage, the Thalassotherapy pool. This time I was actually going to experience the 'health' aspect though – to try out the exercises that Wayne Lèal has been using to train athletes, captains of industry and ordinary people like myself; the Super-Ager programme that works on your body and your mind, promising a better you.

> **"I have tended to procrastinate, when I needed to be more decisive. Now I make decisions and tend to stick by them"**
>
> Helen Sutton

I'd always considered myself relatively fit, because I'm slim (perhaps resting on my laurels a bit), but the two don't necessarily go together. I've always done some sort of exercise, but was never very good at sticking to one thing. Rushing around after small kids was very aerobic and went on for a few years. I played tennis in the B group of the league, until my elbow started hurting too much (it still does if I lift things the wrong way). I tried a dance/exercise class for quite a while – until the teacher got pregnant and had to stop. As for yoga, I'd first started classes years ago in London, but my most vivid memory is not of new positions each week but of prodding my softly snoring friend to wake her up at the end of relaxation time. In Buenos Aires I had been more dedicated; cycling to yoga, meditating and saluting the sun in between classes. Since coming back to the UK, I tried Zumba classes in a fit of enthusiasm and found it fun, but my arm and leg co-ordination was unpredictable, so when I started working, and it (almost) conflicted with work hours, that was all the excuse I needed. I did yoga alone in the privacy of my room, but couldn't tell if my back was straight or my twist was in the right direction. I knew some of my muscles could really do with building up, though - and perhaps my stomach could be a bit less wrinkly.

Turning up the Champneys driveway in Tring was like arriving at a stately home. Swathes of green, a poetic sprinkling of daffodils (I went in the spring) and then the house itself. This whole complex dedicated to pampering and improving yourself?! I was looking forward to this. I know there are members of Champneys, regular weekenders who know the staff by name, but for me it was a new and novel experience. I wasn't here for the pampering though – just the improving part, if the Super-Ager workshop lived up to expectations. I've been told that there were 180 people at Champneys that day; but inside all was serene – people wandering in white bathrobes, no frenetic activity. Just how I thought it should be – sophisticated fitness, no frantic aerobic music or sweaty bodies on show. A brief tour didn't reveal many more of them, though. The gym was deserted, state-of-the-art equipment standing silent. I found a dozen or so in the pool doing an aquaerobics class, but that still left a lot unaccounted for! Perhaps they were all having massages? There are dozens of treatment rooms at Tring offering a myriad of different ways to pamper yourself, not to mention water beds, magazines, hot tub, saunas and steam rooms. An early morning massage would have been quite nice….but no, I concentrated on feeling smug as I made my way to the annex for our workshop – this is a Health Spa, and I was going to get healthy (I know, expecting a lot from a one-day workshop, but no harm in setting your sights high!)

I had heard all the background information and theories from numerous discussions with Wayne himself. His enthusiasm and conviction could persuade the most reluctant of individuals that it is possible to change, and is worth going through the process of deciding you need to alter, fixing a goal and developing a strategy, then doing it. The doing-it-for-long-enough-to-have-a-lasting-effect was apparently the hardest bit, but not a worry for that day. In the workshop we'd be covering the three exercise options expounded by the programme; rebounding, aqua and yoga, using 'repetitions of short sequences of movements, effective without straining the muscles or impacting the joints'...and hopefully setting goals by the end of it. Luckily it turned out there were also pauses worked into the schedule for introductions, explanations, questions, background stories and lunch.

First the introductions – luckily for us we were a small group that day; so it meant that we got more individual attention than usual. Sharing the workshop with me were Gina and Cathy. Gina was a 62-year-old lady from London who had limited mobility due to a hip replacement and a damaged shoulder, recently unpinned, from a bad fall. Her physical problems and her recent and very sudden bereavement had also left her emotionally fragile and with limited confidence re herself as well as her abilities. Physiotherapy had frustrated her – pain blocked many of the movements she was prescribed to do, and a doctor's suggestion that she take a pain-killer and get on with the exercises, had hardly improved her state of mind. She had reached the point where the fear of pain made her shy away from unnecessary movement. Wayne had met her at his talk the previous week, and she had felt an instant empathy, a connection with him. Perhaps since he had suffered injury too, he understood where she was, but he had managed to come through it. He put it to her that very often fear of failure is worse than failure itself. The first step may be the hardest, but once you set out...

Cathy, in contrast, was a 51-year-old who had lived in the US, but was now based in Scotland. Outgoing and enthusiastic, she was at the other end of the fitness spectrum. She and her husband went on cycling trips to far flung destinations once or twice a year, such as through South America or around India, whilst she spent the intervening time working out to keep fit, and had a personal trainer. I was surprised to see her there, but she openly declared that her principal motivation for attending the workshop was curiosity. She had also attended Wayne's talk, was intrigued by the idea of a different and original fitness programme, and wanted to know the 'why' as well as the 'how' for each exercise as we went along. At first glance it looked as if she had already achieved her fitness goal.

It seemed that we couldn't have been three more different ladies, but we were all attending the workshop. That broke the ice and the sense of a common purpose linked us together for the day.

We began with the rebounder: the jumping part of JumpGa; and an explanation of how the weightlessness aspect of bouncing increases its effectiveness. The science behind it all made sense and you wonder why no one has thought of it before – especially since it is so much fun too. Remember bouncing on your bed when you were young? Well, this is almost as good, and you don't have to straighten the sheets afterwards.

We started off just stepping, i.e. pushing the heels down alternately without the feet leaving the surface. It sounds relaxing but it involved balancing too, and we had been told by Wayne to pay attention to our posture all the time, which made me aware how erratic mine was! I corrected so many times it must surely be a reflex action by now. The stepping and bouncing bit was fun; but just when we got the hang of it, he put weights in our hands and we had to run on the spot, lift our arms out in front, bounce whilst holding the weights aloft and do star jumps and squats; each for just a minute at a time.

Remembering to breathe at the same time was my biggest challenge – I was very embarrassed at getting dizzy for a few moments and having to sit instead of jump. It was all short bursts of intense activity, though (the repetition of short sequences that characterises the Super-Ager programme) and then a 'step, breathe and stretch' break in between.

Cathy and I managed this part quite well, once we got the hang of staying in the middle of the rebounder (and if you overlook my little dizzy spell). Gina though, was very unsure of her balance. At Wayne's suggestion she had placed her rebounder at the edge of the room; and kept one hand on the wall all through the exercise to steady, or reassure, herself.

Wayne was beside us throughout: a voice giving encouragement, bits of 'gentle' correction and the odd annoying comment: 'watch your posture…keep your heels pushing downwards…don't round your shoulders… you can run faster & squat lower…don't slow down!'

Then came the pool exercises: Kun-Aqua! The aquaerobics class participants were long gone, and there were only two or three swimmers doing a few leisurely lengths. Our first task was to walk in a straight line very slowly through the water. Here Gina had her moment. She surprised us all, except Wayne – who seemed to know her strengths and weaknesses better than she did herself. Her weak hip and shoulder were supported in the water and she ploughed through it ahead of us, in a straight line. Cathy and I, in contrast, were floored by this simple task. Cathy set out impulsively to complete the exercise quickly, but couldn't keep in a straight line. I was also pulled to one side by the water and had trouble with the precision of the steps in the water. We had assumed that it was easy and hence didn't immediately engage our concentration. Any movement was intensified by the pressure of the water, which itself set out to unbalance us – and we found ourselves relearning how to walk. It was okay though, we were starting to realise that it was acceptable to be 'not good' at something and to have to start learning anew.

I actually found going backwards through the water a little easier to control, which I thought must make me somehow unusual (like my left-handedness), but apparently it's just that you have a different centre of gravity and better balance with your bottom (i.e. a heavier part of you) leading.

Perhaps because we were a small group, perhaps because we had realised that each of us had strengths and weaknesses and hence something new to learn – by the time the arm exercises came round, we were united, initially in battle against the pool. I was intrigued that splayed fingers of the hand offered greater resistance against the water, as long as they are kept tensed. The whisper between us of 'no floppy hands' provoked schoolgirl giggles throughout the rest of the day.

That was our morning, and we moved on to the restaurant. Lunch isn't really part of the workshop itself but, aside from being a very tempting buffet in Champneys restaurant, it gave us a chance to talk around the sessions and about ourselves.

Gina told us how she fell and hurt her shoulder, and then moved on to stories of other places and spas she had visited. Those coincided with some of Cathy's cycling trips to far-flung destinations, which in turn led into a discussion of my travels and time in South America, compared to Cathy's trip through it.

I also finally discovered where all those Champneys guests had been hanging out between treatments. Gym empty, pool empty, restaurant full…white-robed figures were seated at almost every table, or perusing the buffet. Perhaps they had come on a weekend, all-inclusive package and were taking the 'I've paid for it so I'm going to have it' attitude to lunch. I don't blame them – it was good: a buffet spread to rival the five-star hotels, but all healthily prepared, nothing fried (although, to my delight, the BBC recently told me that fried eggs are okay because they don't absorb the oil) and beautiful colour combinations, since every good chef knows that presentation is an art in itself. Apparently they do also have a super light menu and even a separate dining area if you don't want to risk the temptation to revisit. I could have gone round several times, but worked hard on my 'holier than thou' feeling: eating a small salad, trying not to think about the massage rooms and knowing that I had spent my morning doing something great for my body.

After our light lunch and discussions, Cathy left for a brisk walk whilst I joined Gina at her pace for a more leisurely stroll, finding time for a coffee and a chat. Then it was back to the workshop for after lunch stretching, and yoga.

This was where we discovered that whilst we thought we already did yoga, we weren't really very good at it. Or to be more specific: our postures could be better and our joints more supple. My hips, for example, are too stiff – hence my back doesn't tilt from them, it bends and is sort of banana shaped, when it shouldn't be.

We learnt a variation on the sun salutation and then took to the wall, i.e. doing postures against it to check our alignment; seeing which bits touched in a straight line, or didn't when they should do.

The end of the official workshop was a discussion – stories from Wayne about his experiences, analyses and admissions from ourselves about our goals: what we had learnt about ourselves from the day, what we could take away, use and adopt in order to build a strategy of our own; to arrive where we wanted to be this time next year.

Wayne offered us his own evaluation of where each of us was:

Cathy – so energetic, she is always moving, always needs to be in motion – yet not necessarily the most efficient activity for her body. In between her frenetic bursts of activity she needs to practise mindfulness and simply slow down a little to bring her body into balance.

Gina – in her fragile physical and emotional state, had surprised herself regarding the elements that she was able to excel in. She had benefited enormously from having a sense of empathy, that someone sympathised and understood what she was experiencing; which would hopefully help with her next stage of physical recuperation.

Helen (me) - so full of plans and ambitions, she had always tended to start projects and make plans but given up when the going got tough. A lack of self-esteem meant she simply assumed she would fail. For her, taking on a programme like Super-Ager offered the chance to follow a set of steps towards a goal, changing little things to improve the big picture.

I, for one, left fired with enthusiasm and a renewed sense of self confidence. Those white-robed guests didn't know what they had missed out on. Wayne had given me the feeling that I could achieve wonderful things, if I really wanted to. I told him, and myself, that I wanted to feel fitter, develop more muscles and have fewer wrinkly bits; that I will make the changes I need to get there. That commitment – voicing aloud what you aim to do – is important. Once you've told someone else, there is a consequence to success or failure.

So it becomes a challenge for me now. I didn't specify how much fitter, or how many fewer wrinkles – but I know how I want to feel. If I fall by the wayside I will feel I have let Wayne down, but more importantly I'll have let myself down. So…I'm setting my alarm clock a little earlier, doing my yoga poses, trying to be mindful and kind to myself, making my healthy smoothie for breakfast, cycling everywhere I can (I know that wasn't in the Super-Ager Programme but it is still deemed very healthy) – and deciding which rebounder to buy.

I'd like to go back in a year; to do it all again and see how different I feel… and perhaps try a massage…

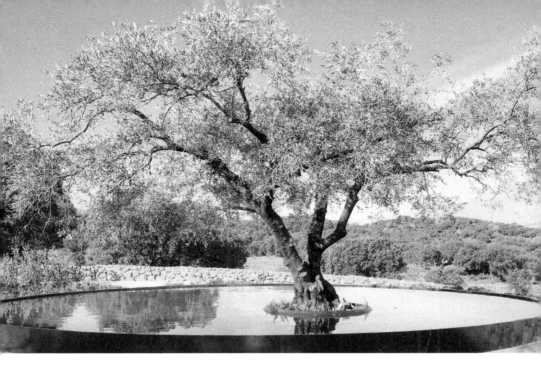

## ANN: FITNESS AS A HABIT

Ann is a cycling and mountain biking enthusiast; spending weekends in the saddle with like-minded friends. She is also a club member at Champneys and uses it as her local gym for cross training.

*"Fitness is such an important part of my life now"*

So why is she here, in the stories of 'converts to the Super-Ager programme'? It sounds as if she already reached termination on the wheel of behavioural change. If she is fit enough to cycle for whole weekends and has an established exercise routine; surely she can't have much more of a goal to achieve? Wrong! Almost everyone has a weakness lurking somewhere, some physical problem holding them back, or an aspect of their training or their mindset that could be just that little bit better.

The advert for Wayne's weekly motivational talk at Champneys caught Ann's eye at a time when she was stagnating in her exercise routine. Serious knee problems were preventing her from running, so she was looking for a substitute exercise to fit into her cross training programme.

The serious knee problem is osteoarthritis. Surgery has been carried out on her right knee, releasing the tendons so that the patella is no longer catching on the femoral surface – and hopefully avoiding further wearing of it, since the only other option now (according to the surgeon) is a unilateral knee replacement. According to Ann herself 'They creak when I move – which is a bit strange but it helps remind me to take care of them, to be a bit more mindful!' The theory/hope is that, by keeping the muscles strong around the problem area, she can limit further damage.

At the initial talk, Wayne was apparently full of his usual charisma and held the room spellbound throughout his lecture. Ann was sufficiently impressed and moved on from there to the workshop a few weeks later. Again Wayne was a fantastic role model: 'uncompromising, tough and professional; but with a wicked sense of humour.'

As for the exercises themselves? The two aspects to the programme are JumpGa and Kun-Aqua. There are various exercises within each area but none impact on the joints and all challenge coordination of the body and the mind. People come to the workshop at all sorts of different stages in the process of change, some foundering and needing direction, others already heading along a path. Ann, as she said, was already committed to exercise and looking for a slightly different direction – an alternative to incorporate into her routine to inspire her, rather than needing inspiration per se.

Two other attendees at this particular workshop were also club members. Ladies of a similar age and mindset to Ann, they were looking to alter their training a little, hoping to find something that would fit into the limited time they have available yet still be a good all round exercise regime that wouldn't hurt or damage a 50-plus body. Another couple taking part were a little older, citing their main sport and exercise as golf. They didn't attend Champneys regularly for exercise but each had knee and back problems and were looking for an alternative exercise option.

The best gauge of the workshop's success is perhaps not what happens on the day itself, but rather what people take away from it; what they aim to practise and include in their lives from there on in.

Ann herself cites fitness as being 'such an important part of my life now'. She goes once a week to the gym, and includes a rebounding session in her workout. Rebounding aggravated her knees during the initial workshop session, but building up slowly, with weekly practice, they have more or less adapted. Now it firmly hits the spot as a cardiovascular workout as beneficial as running – but one that decreases shock and stress to the joints. As Wayne said 'With rebounding all of the muscles in your body are activated as they adjust to the increased gravitational pull.' As Ann points out, 'The really great thing is the simultaneous upper body workout (an area where women are typically weaker) that you can get from using weights whilst on the rebounder. It makes it a sort of multitasking exercise!' It also helped to strengthen her right shoulder again, dislocated when she fell off her bike.

Once a week she also goes to the pool: swimming lengths and then following the sequence of walking, arm and leg exercises shown by Wayne at the Super-Ager workshop. According to Wayne, they move a fixed amount of resistance through a specific range of motion and so give a consistent controlled exercise – not forgetting that the water protects the joints by reducing impact. According to Ann, though, as well as practising these in the pool she found a great knock on effect. After the workshop there is always an intriguing element of mix and match for anyone who is already exercising in some shape or form – discovering how the exercises learnt in the Super-Ager programme meld in with established workouts or into daily life to make something just that little bit better. For Ann, by far the best example came from the pool exercises. 'Just' walking through the water means having to engage your core strength to achieve control and balance, counteracting the pull and pressure of the water. She translated it to the initial force required on a bike to start pedalling uphill and said, 'It was quite a revelation how changing my posture and then engaging my core muscles could help so significantly.' Wayne does mention in his talks how small incremental changes will build up into something more.

The last 'once a week' is yoga. 'Each pose of the sequence requires an integration of focus, strength and fluidity – challenging coordination and concentration'. After practising Hatha yoga for quite a while, Ann is now trying the challenge of Bikram yoga (aka hot yoga: a form of yoga synthesised from Hatha yoga techniques; consisting of a fixed sequence of postures, practised in a heated and humid room) and says, 'I'm really starting to feel the benefits throughout my body. I think I might even be getting a little better at it each week!'

Aside from the physical aspects, Ann's mindset has adapted in balance with the new exercises. She has replaced packets of crisps with smoothies and is eating less junk food all round. A new exercise routine seems to have extended to a new routine full stop; a more holistic approach to the whole general issue of wellbeing.

Ann certainly plans to carry on with what she's started, and wishes that Wayne would do a follow up to the workshop: '…to help those who are still practising the programme, to get their techniques checked or modified; and perhaps be taught a few new exercises to work into their routines.'

At the time of the workshop, Ann admitted that she weighed 9 stone 10 lb, against the 9 stone that she had clocked in at for the past 10 years. Since then, though, between sensible eating and her newly jigged exercise routine; she has lost half a stone and is back to her 'ideal weight'. Not only that but Ann reckons she is back to being as fit now as she was five years ago. That is quite an accolade if you think of her knees and the challenge of sticking to a rigorous exercise plan as the years go by; and even more impressive given her own description of herself a few years back as '…a 20 a day smoker at the age of 30, doing no exercise whatsoever; except walking to the pub.'

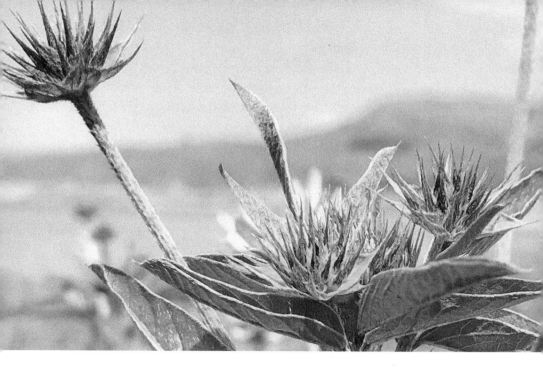

## SUSAN RODWAY QC

Among Wayne's past pupils is Susan Rodway QC. Renowned for her advocacy skills and with over 12 years' experience acting as leading counsel, she found the inspiration and strength in Wayne's training to rebuild her life after a 'rough patch'. This is her 'Wayne story'.

*'Super-Ager Fitness is not just about moving your body – it's about strengthening your mind and spirit.'*

I first met Wayne Lèal in 2011, through the yoga classes he was giving in Fulham. I had done some research on Wayne and was very impressed with his CV. It was also unusual at that time to find a male yoga instructor, the majority being female. My curiosity was piqued and I went along just to see.

I had attended a few yoga classes on and off in the past but regarded myself as an almost complete novice.

In 2011 I was 56 years old and in the throes of an acrimonious divorce. My husband of 20 years had walked out on me, unexpectedly, in 2009 and then started proceedings to attempt to obtain financial support. He had removed all of his financial contribution to the household overnight and had cut off all contact with our four children. I was struggling to maintain the household and stay on top of my career as well as deal with the litigation and court hearings; which I was running myself in order to save costs.

I will never forget the introduction to that first class. Wayne introduced himself and then told us an analogy about leaving all of our baggage that was weighing us down at the door of the studio. We could pick up our 'baggage' again at the end of the class; but for this one hour we were to let go of all our problems and give our total concentration to ourselves ... to be the best that we could be.

This was an epiphany for me. I had been to counselling and psychotherapy. I had tried formal gym classes. I had taken long walks. Nothing had struck a chord in the way that Wayne's simple introduction did that day. I was totally hooked.

The actual class itself was also a revelation. Although I was a complete beginner, the class was aimed at all levels. Wayne reiterated strongly that 'bending yourself into a pretzel' was not the aim of yoga. I realised that in so many walks of life there are those continually trying to prove themselves better than others. We are never better than all the others. Showing off or needing admiration is merely a demonstration of our own inner lack of security.

The injury that I was subconsciously seeking to heal was, in fact, my broken sense of self. Through Wayne's classes I opened myself up to self-exploration and started my journey back to self-appreciation. I gained not only my physical but my mental fitness... and I rediscovered my sense of fun.

After this I was a Wayne regular. I followed him everywhere and took private lessons as well. I was probably one of the early guinea pigs for

Super-Ager, in that the programme he developed with me was based on his training of athletes (I hasten to say that I am NOT one of those!). I progressed to aqua exercise on top of formal gym/ weights work and yoga; and then this evolved into the Super-Ager programme of aqua / yoga and rebounding.

Having become an afficionado, I now practise the programme on my own. I travel extensively and cannot take my rebounder when I am abroad, but I have developed the habit of doing at least one yoga practice every single day... even if it is as short as 10 or 15 minutes. At least three times a week I do a combined rebounder and yoga practice for about an hour and, whenever I can, I add in the pool work.

I am now 61 years old but my level of fitness is far superior to that of when I was in my thirties. I have old injuries from riding, skiing and motorcycling; but can honestly say that I now pay no attention to them. The pain that they used to cause me is a thing of the past.

Psychologically I have moved on and am fulfilled and happy. The darks days of the divorce are long past and I have a new partner and a new family (with two step sons) I am literally reborn and starting my life again.

Thank you so much Wayne.

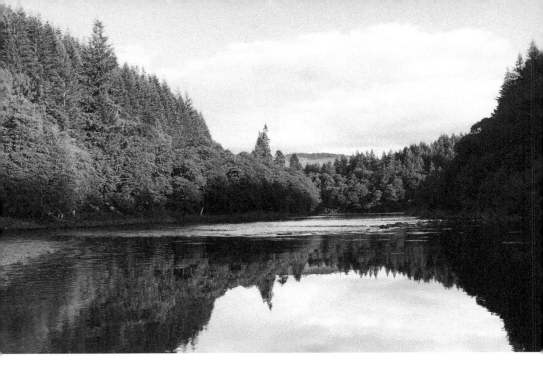

## CHERYL MORLEY – A WAY TO WALK

I should sum up a little, and explain just where my life had gone before meeting Wayne. In February 2013 I had a hip replacement operation that I initially recovered from reasonably well, but then began experiencing pain again. On investigation, it transpired that a piece of bone had splintered away during the operation and had become lodged in the muscles, hence the pain. The only solution offered, apart from more surgery, was physiotherapy. I persevered with this for a while, but got nowhere fast and it was extremely painful. I tried all manner of different therapies but nothing really worked. I also went swimming regularly and used the running machine at the gym (not running, just walking). Eventually, after about a year it did seem to be easing somewhat but was still not totally 100% right.

*'In a nutshell, I feel
I owe so much to
Wayne. It's as if I
have got my life back
since meeting him...'*

Cheryl Morley

Then in August 2014 I contracted staphylococcus which unfortunately went undiagnosed for two weeks, by which time it had got a complete hold of me. To cut a long and painful story short, I underwent two knee operations, a spine operation and two more hip replacement operations to get rid of the infection and was on IV antibiotics for several months. Then I also fractured my femur to boot. Needless to say I was in a pretty poor way; both physically and mentally.

When we went to Cyprus in June 2015, it was our first proper holiday for over a year, simply because I had been so unwell and unable to travel anywhere. The Anassa Hotel in Latchi is fantastic, but it is spread over such a large area that, whilst absolutely beautiful; there is a lot of walking involved to get anywhere. To be quite honest; my heart sank when we arrived because I didn't know how I was going to cope. I think it must have been serendipity, that day when we met Wayne in the pool at the spa. Up until then, walking was very painful and quite frankly I felt every bit and more of my 60 years, which depressed me no end!

The Kun-Aqua exercises he taught me to do in the pool have quite literally worked a miracle – I feel transformed. Even after the first session I could feel a big difference and was moving much more easily. I sensed that he really empathised with me, because of some of his injuries in the past, and could understand at least a part of what I was going through. We have also bought a rebounder to use at home and I have tried to continue the JumpGa exercises we were shown on that too, although my husband uses it more than I do. I enjoy the water exercises most of all and combine them with swimming at least 10 to 15 lengths of the pool – by the end of which I really feel I have had a good workout; but pain free!

I saw my hip consultant when we returned from Cyprus, and he quite literally could not believe how well I was walking. The last time I saw him, and it had only been at the end of April, I was still on two walking sticks. Of course, I told him all about Wayne Lèal and his wondrous exercise programme.

The Super-Ager programme is absolutely fantastic and I can't sing Wayne's praises highly enough. I should point out that I don't really like exercising in general and never have done, but I realise that it is necessary; particularly as one becomes older. I do really like being in a pool, though, and can honestly say I enjoy the water exercises – particularly loving the way I feel when I have finished them. The buoyancy of the water supports me, meaning I can move more easily without stressing my joints.

I exercise to keep in shape generally, but mainly for mobility. If you are really overweight I don't believe that exercise is a substitute for dieting, but in any case I don't consider my exercise regime anywhere near rigorous enough to reduce my weight.

Back just before Christmas I caught flu; and my illness, combined with winter, meant that I didn't go to the pool for two or three months. I guess in the model of changing behaviour that Wayne told me about, I would be classed as having relapsed. I have started going back again now though, and for the past couple of months have been gradually building up my strength. I am afraid that it is also harder to maintain enthusiasm in the winter, despite the gym club being well heated, especially when there seem to be a lot of swimming classes taking place at various times of day. I have finally worked out a timetable that suits me and avoids them, though, so have no more excuses. The best exercise periods for me are when we holiday abroad and I can use the hotel pool two or three times a day for several weeks. This builds up the benefit for me, and I really see the difference in my mobility.

I have recently added acupuncture to my 'health regime', which is also offering some relief from the pain and I'm going to try yoga in the near future, as another element from Wayne's Super-Ager programme.

I feel transformed by everything that Wayne has taught me…and still find it hard to believe that I could see such amazing benefits in such a short space of time!

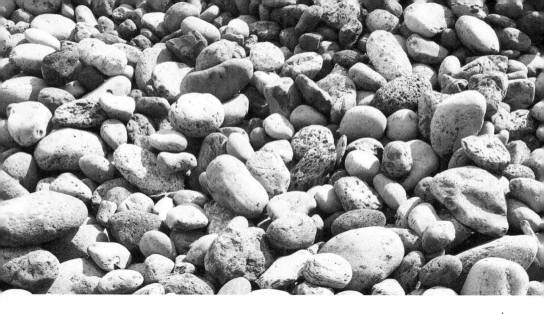

## CLAIRE WEINBERG – BEATING CANCER

Claire was diagnosed with breast cancer in August 2008, having moved to America 12 years before. She had first started training with Wayne in 1992, and it was then that he had first started designing his revolutionary workout. It was this that Claire felt helped save her life after she called on his expertise again.

Claire said: "I was in an emotionally abusive and very unhappy marriage. I had no support network after what was a devastating diagnosis.

Wayne went through all of the motivational lessons with me that he had taught me from the beginning. I would be feeling at my lowest, in the fight of my life, and I would hear Wayne's voice – pushing me on. It was telling me I was in control of my body and that I could beat anything – even cancer."

Claire went on to say: "Wayne absolutely helped me beat cancer. I knew from the training I had done with him that I could succeed and I was resilient. He was the support that I carried with me, because I felt alone emotionally."

Communications and marketing manager Claire – who ended her marriage after her cancer battle – now enjoys extreme sports with son Gabe, 13. "I want to be able to keep up with him. Thanks to Wayne, I can."

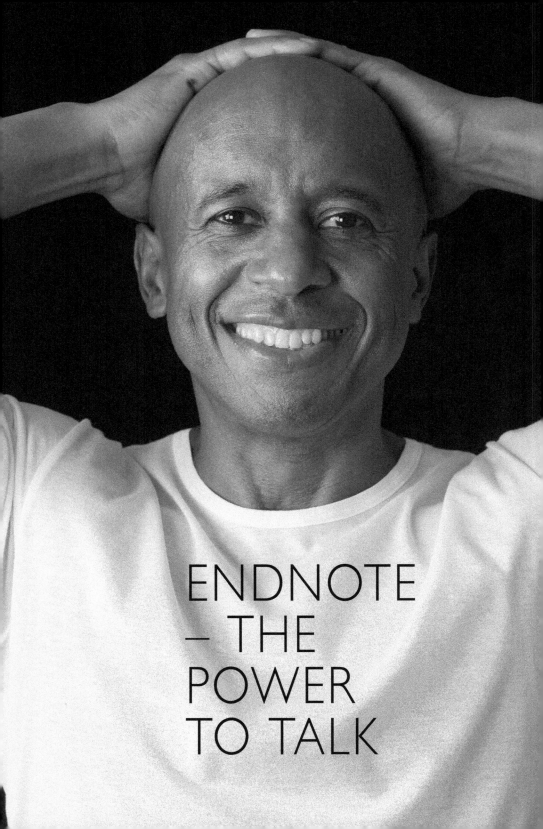

ENDNOTE
– THE
POWER
TO TALK

WAYNE IS NOT 'just' a Health Coach'. He is an empathetic and inspirational speaker – as attested by many of the stories in this book. Darren Barker was inspired by Wayne's words as much as his fitness programme, as was Ryan Bertrand and many of the clients who have come to Wayne's classes through attending his motivational talks. He is also an excellent keynote speaker.

A keynote speaker is an expert in a particular field who can relate their content to improving businesses and inspiring staff. The best among them are able to capture the essence of a meeting and in turn capture the attention of the audience. As a keynote speaker Wayne's talks are an inspirational odyssey. He likens the art of being an inspirational speaker to that of being a great storyteller – recounting a series of experiences that give knowledge or understanding to someone.

His secret, he says, is confidence – that 'simple' foundation for everything in life – that intangible thing which makes the difference between feeling weak and feeling powerful.

It's true, we all need it – to be convinced that we can be and do a lot more than we are being or doing right now, if we just try. With that confidence we present a different face to the world, affecting how others see and perceive us both socially and in business. If you can see the path ahead of you and feel yourself to be unstoppable, that confidence will push aside almost any obstacle in your way.

His childhood was a struggle but with tenacity and a little inspiration of his own he managed to turn adversity into opportunity. From a racial attack in his teens, leaving him with a fractured skull, he moved on to be who he is. Looking back, but without putting a label on things, and refusing to be embittered by the experience, he says that the attack made him identify more clearly what he wanted and how he wanted to live his life.

Envy is another natural condition that has deep biological roots and can affect our lives according to how we deal with it. Wayne experienced it, in large quantities, as a boy walking home past the beautiful houses in

Chelsea. That level of social comparison, of inequality, always made him evaluate his own position on the bottom rung of the ladder; and what would it take to adjust it.

For many people it's the absence of belief in themselves and their abilities that directly affects where they are going, who they are and how they do everything in life.

At some stage in most people's lives they have needed to conquer this lack of confidence. How did Wayne do it? There is no magic pill, but the overwhelming scientific evidence of the mental benefits of physical exercise keep stacking up. He says that when working with clients he can clearly see how physical transformation brings about an increased level of confidence. There is a mental high that comes with feeling physically fit. Look good, feel good.

It is true. Confidence is not just in the mind – you can convince others from the outside – and yourself too. During Wayne's workshop and talk he can be heard saying: 'How you walk affects how you feel, and in turn how others perceive you. Walking slouched with your head down can make you feel low and sends out a negative impression to the people around you. Instead, walk proud and tall: when you move with purpose it makes a world of difference.'

On any given day in London there are probably at least 100 speakers at various events around the city. Every single medium or large-sized business has an annual meeting, and so does every single association. Interestingly, but not really surprisingly, Wayne's keynote talks have been primarily to female audiences. His words empower them and instil the confidence they need to thrive in a male-dominated environment.

As a keynote speaker, Wayne is always being hired by new organisations and some will bring him back a second or even a third time. Upon first invitation he spends a lot of time researching the companies, developing his content and building his keynote programme to showcase his message and delivery. He has never taken a professional speaker's course, saying: 'I'm sure they're excellent but I really do understand how to deliver a good speech.' He speaks from experience; offering himself as proof that what he suggests actually works, and the anecdotes in his speeches are real ones, from his own life.

Among those who ask him back over and over is Champneys Health Spa in Tring. For over a year Wayne has been a regular speaker there, inspiring clients to instigate a change in their lives, advocating health and fitness as a springboard for improvement in all areas of life. His success lies in the fact that he is leading, as all the great leaders in history have done, by example. He is not merely telling his audience to 'do this' or 'do that': he is the physical and mental epitome of what he teaches – 'do what I have done and see where it will get you'. His genuine desire to impart knowledge and to help others to increase their confidence in their own self-image is the end result of his own journey of discovery and makes him an inspiring teacher. People are caught up in his experiences and inspired by his conviction.

There are four general categories of keynote speaking: leadership, overcoming adversity, motivation and inspiration. Leadership and overcoming adversity speak for themselves. Motivation is the act of convincing people to do things that they already know they should be doing. Wayne falls into the inspiration category and considers it by far the most exciting. He says, 'I enjoy inspiring people to do things that they had never thought of doing until they heard my speech!'

The term 'keynote' comes from the practice among cappella singers of playing a note before singing, to determine the key in which the song will be performed…Hence a keynote speaker worth his or her salt will lead the audience down a chosen path.

When we know and value who we are, it manifests itself in the form of a great feeling about ourselves. This confidence helps us go on to make better choices and better decisions in private and business lives. In making these better choices and better decisions, we go on to be happier at home and more productive at work – a much improved life all round.

As a global teacher Wayne is aware that it doesn't matter what country, organisation or spa he visits, confidence is a problem that people of all ages, genders and races can have. It is very apparent that everything is based on our self-confidence and that it is extremely important in every aspect of our lives, yet so many people struggle to find it.

When we are born our confidence is perfectly intact but diminishes during our childhood. Everyone loses a little of it but sometimes it is down to circumstances, or parents placing too much academic pressure on their children, or criticising when they make mistakes, fail, misbehave, get into trouble, or admit to feeling guilty, or doing things they are ashamed of. In the wrong circumstance, sentiment can be seen as a weakness and criticism of it lead to self-doubt.

Sometimes confidence is born from a believed situation rather than a real one, but can serve just as strongly in someone's life nonetheless. Wayne speaks of his son JJ having an interview for a secondary school. He told him even if you don't know the answer to a question give them an answer, guessing something is better than no answer at all. On the day JJ was asked a series of religious questions that he was expected to know from his Sunday school attendance. The problem was that he went to 6 pm mass (missing Sunday school) because he played for a successful football team every Sunday morning. JJ did as his father said and answered with confidence, to the point that Wayne was really impressed. At the end, as JJ and his mother exited the room, Wayne asked the teacher quietly 'How did he do?' and the teacher said that he got most of the questions wrong. But when Wayne met JJ and his mother outside and asked: 'How do you think you did?' JJ replied, 'I didn't have a clue what she was asking me, but I remembered what you said and gave her an answer.' That little experiment worked because JJ is now a confident young man, very rarely fazed by anyone or anything.

The best business successes first existed in the confidence of those who created them. Wayne knows that, as a Keynote Speaker, you are hired to speak at an event, to inspire others. The only thing you're selling is your message; though, if you try to sell an actual product or specific service, you would never be asked back.

Wayne's first corporate keynote speaker event with 100+ attendees was a nerve-racking experience. Fortunately for Wayne, though, he has the two vital ingredients that make him popular onstage: inspiration and humour. People learn when they laugh.

Wayne always closes his talk with an inspirational invitation to the guests. 'Give what I said a go. I promise you it will help you to create more confidence in your life and – best of all – it will help you to get from where you are now to where you want to be in your life.'

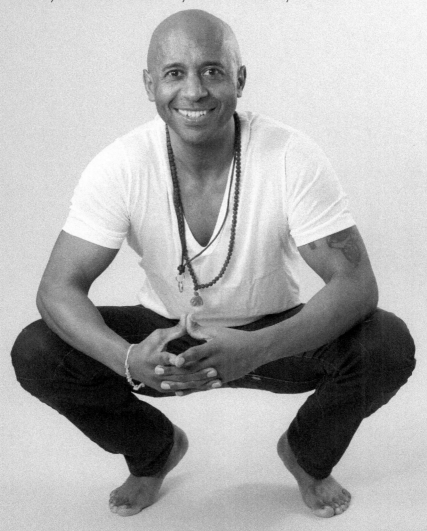

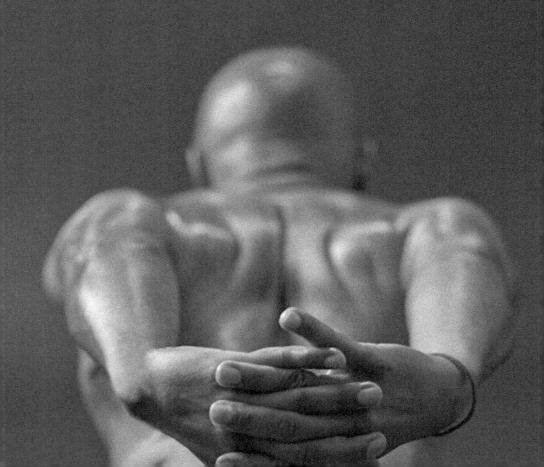

"Question assumed beliefs about ageing. And take the radical leap needed to become a Super-Ager."

*Wayne Lèal*

9 781912 969586